Urinary Continence and Sexual Function After Robotic Prostatectomy, Radiation, and Novel Therapies

Sanjay Razdan • Shirin Razdan
Editors

Urinary Continence and Sexual Function After Robotic Prostatectomy, Radiation, and Novel Therapies

Second Edition

Springer

Editors
Sanjay Razdan
International Robotic Institute for
Prostate Cancer
Doral, FL, USA

Shirin Razdan
Miami Robotic Surgery at the
Comprehensive Urologic Surgery Institute
Miami, FL, USA

ISBN 978-3-031-64244-9 ISBN 978-3-031-64245-6 (eBook)
https://doi.org/10.1007/978-3-031-64245-6

This Springer imprint is published by the registered company Springer Nature Switzerland AG
The registered company address is: Gewerbestrasse 11, 6330 Cham, Switzerland

Preface

This book represents the second edition in our series examining functional outcomes after prostate cancer treatment. Our first edition, published in 2016, was titled *Urinary Continence and Sexual Function After Robotic Radical Prostatectomy* and featured chapters written by the world's premier robotic prostate surgeons on how to optimize outcomes post-robotic prostatectomy (RALP). Now almost 8 years later, with a lot more data and techniques described in the literature, we present our new textbook titled *Urinary Continence and Sexual Function After Robotic Prostatectomy, Radiation, and Novel Therapies*. In this edition, we go beyond RALP and delve into outcomes post-radiation, brachytherapy, and focal therapy as well.

Over time we realized that the future of prostate cancer care is in precision medicine. With novel tools, technologies, and therapies in practice, we owe it to our patients and our colleagues to effectively discuss all the available treatment options and their ramifications. Optimizing outcomes is not simply radical extirpation of tumor but rather taking both patient and tumor factors into consideration to devise a treatment plan that is most beneficial in terms of cancer cure and functional outcomes of continence and erectile function.

Our book is divided into 13 chapters. Since the foundation of all prostate-related treatment is in the intricate neurovascular anatomy of the pelvis, we begin our book with a thorough discussion of the anatomy of the prostate, the cavernous nerves, the urethral sphincter complex, and the supporting musculofascial layers. This book then continues with preoperative assessment of prostate cancer and methods to optimize urinary continence and erectile function prior to treatment. Subsequent chapters detail intraoperative and postoperative techniques to improve functional outcomes, including a chapter and video accompaniment on salvage RALP and other challenging clinical scenarios in RALP. We conclude this book with a discussion on radiation therapy and focal therapy for prostate cancer and their effects on erectile function and urinary continence. Finally, the closing chapter is on the future of prostate cancer care, with an overview of precision prostatectomy, artificial intelligence, and targeted immunotherapy options for patients. At the end of each chapter is a "Take Home Message" from us, the editors. These are succinct pearls that we believe the reader should keep in mind while studying the textbook.

It is a great honor to serve as co-editor of this book that my father brought to fruition for the first time many years ago. Through residency and fellowship, I have seen the dynamics of prostate cancer diagnosis and treatment change. Patients are more well-informed and asking incisive questions regarding their individual oncological risks and treatment-specific outcomes. As such, we strove to expand upon our prior work to address these new patient-specific concerns while still maintaining the core ethos of our book: maximizing functional outcomes regardless of treatment modality. We invite readers to delve into our book as we believe there is something to take away for urologists in every stage of their career.

Throughout robotic surgeons' training, video-based learning is the cornerstone to reinforce the skills that the surgeon practices in the operating room, and we encourage trainees to utilize these resources in the same way. The video accompaniments to our book serve to supplement the text and provide greater in-depth descriptions of surgical techniques described in the bodies of the chapters. At the end of the day, better surgical outcomes are guaranteed by better and more prepared surgeons. Better outcomes of radiation and focal therapies are enabled by well-studied practitioners.

On behalf of my co-editor Dr. Sanjay Razdan, I'd like to thank the authors who so graciously contributed to our second edition. Some of the authors are individuals whom I had the pleasure to work with over the past few years, while others are some whom I admire greatly from afar. The field of prostate cancer care is truly collaborative, and none of this work could have been done without the help of a team of surgeons and scientists eager to push the frontiers of urology forward.

We hope you enjoy this textbook. We took great pains to revamp it and make it even more relevant to current practice. The videos that accompany the book should not be ignored, for they may even better show techniques explained in the chapters. Please do not hesitate to reach out to any of the authors or editors should you wish to discuss any of these concepts further. We are all motivated to improve the care rendered to our patients, and teaching and sharing knowledge is fundamental to that vision.

All our best.

Doral, FL, USA Shirin Razdan
Doral, FL, USA Sanjay Razdan

Contents

Anatomic Foundations and Physiology of Erectile Function and Urinary Continence

1

Adriana M. Pedraza, Raghav Gupta, Manish Choudhary, Dhruti Patel, and Ash Tewari

Anatomical Principles and Physiology of Erectile Function

Penile erection is a complex neuroanatomical and physiological phenomenon. To comprehend this process, it is important to examine the anatomy and physiology of the penis. The penis comprises three primary parts: the glans, the penile shaft, and the root. The glans is the bulbous expansion located at the distal end of the penis, primarily composed of the corpus spongiosum. It is densely innervated and considered the most sensitive part of the penis. The penile shaft is composed of three erectile tissues: two corpora cavernosa and one corpus spongiosum. Each corpora cavernosa is located on the dorsolateral part of the penile shaft and is surrounded by a fascial layer called the tunica albuginea. The tunica albuginea is a bilayer structure consisting of inner circular and outer longitudinal layers, primarily composed of elastin and collagenous tissue fibers. Its main function is to provide strength to the penile corporal bodies and contribute to the maintenance of penile rigidity during erection [1].

Running between the two layers of the tunica albuginea are the emissary or tunical veins. These veins play a role in erection by getting compressed during engorgement. This compression prevents the outflow of blood from the penile shaft, contributing to the rigidity of the erect penis. Within the corporal bodies, there are smooth muscle fibers and spongiosal arteries. The smooth muscle fibers facilitate the relaxation necessary to increase the blood flow, and the spongiosal arteries supply the penile tissues with oxygenated blood. Beyond the tunica albuginea, the penile shaft is covered by additional fascial layers known as Buck's fascia and Dartos fascia [1, 2].

A. M. Pedraza (✉) · R. Gupta · M. Choudhary · D. Patel · A. Tewari
Department of Urology, Icahn School of Medicine at Mount Sinai, New York City, NY, USA
e-mail: Raghav.gupta@mountsinai.org; Manish.Choudhary@mountsinai.org; Dhruti.patel@mountsinai.org; Ash.tewari@mountsinai.org

S. Razdan, S. Razdan (eds.), *Urinary Continence and Sexual Function After Robotic Prostatectomy, Radiation, and Novel Therapies*,
https://doi.org/10.1007/978-3-031-64245-6_1

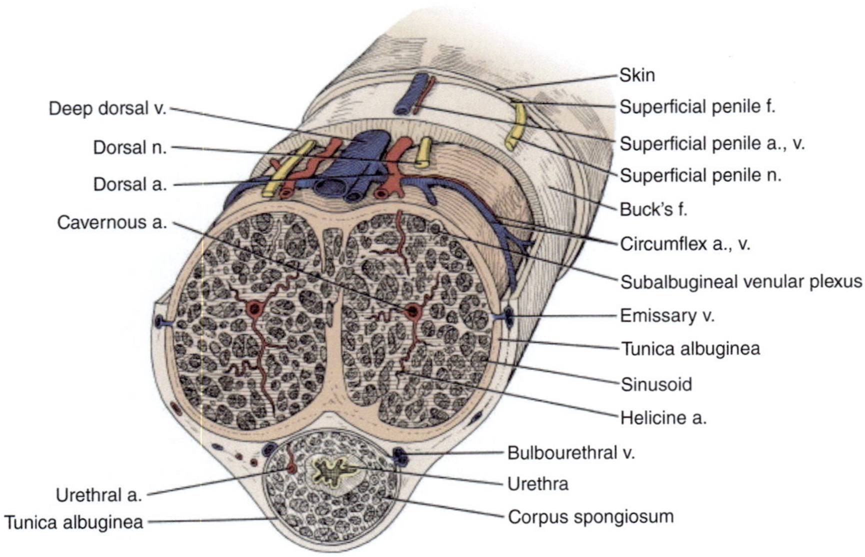

Fig. 1.1 Cross-sectional anatomy of the penis. The penis is composed of three cylindrical masses of the cavernous tissue bound together by the fibrous tissue and covered with the skin. Two of the masses are lateral and are known as the corpus cavernosum; the third is median and is termed the corpus spongiosum. The location of arteries, veins, and urethra are depicted. (Reprinted from MacLennan [25], copyright © 2012, with permission from Elsevier)

The corpus spongiosum is situated on the ventral part of the penile shaft and houses the penile urethra, which allows for the passage of urine and semen during ejaculation.

The root of the penis encompasses the most proximal section and comprises the crura and the bulb of the penis, as well as the ischiocavernosus and bulbocavernosus muscles. The bulb of the penis refers to the proximal dilated part of the spongiosa, while the crura of the penis indicate the proximal dilated part of the corporal bodies, which insert near the inferior pubic bony ramus [1, 3].

The bulbospongiosus and ischiocavernosus muscles play a crucial role in the maintenance of penile rigidity. They compress the bulb of the penis, the spongiosa, and the deep dorsal veins, effectively retaining blood within the penile shaft. This compression helps sustain an erect state of the penis (Fig. 1.1).

Penile Vascular Supply

The arterial supply to the penis is derived from the internal pudendal artery, which is a branch of the internal iliac artery. The internal pudendal artery gives rise to three terminal arteries: the cavernosal artery, dorsal penile artery, and bulbourethral artery. The cavernosal artery runs along the dorsal aspect of the cavernosa. It gives off branches known as helicine arteries, which supply blood to the cavernosal sinusoids, ultimately contributing to penile erection [4].

The venous drainage of the penis involves the superficial, intermediate, and deep dorsal veins. The superficial veins drain the penile skin and travel above Buck's fascia to join the superficial dorsal vein of the penis. The intermediate veins run beneath Buck's fascia and are responsible for draining the glans and the penile shaft. This includes the dorsal vein and the circumflex veins, which play an important role in penile tumescence and the overall venous drainage process. The deep venous system comprises the cavernosal veins, which drain proximally into the internal pudendal vein [1].

Physiology of Penile Erection

Penile erection is a complex physiological response involving coordinated interactions among the penile vasculature, nervous system, and penile tissue. The initiation of sexual response begins in the forebrain and hypothalamus, which activate the central pathways. From there, the neuronal impulses are transmitted through both autonomic and somatomotor pathways [2].

The autonomic pathways, located in the thoracolumbar and sacral segments, along with the somatomotor pathways, play a crucial role in transmitting the neuronal signals. The cavernosal nerves are responsible for relaying the signal to the cavernous penile tissue. This leads to the vasodilation of cavernosal arteries and the relaxation of smooth muscle fibers within the cavernosa [5].

Concurrently, somatomotor stimulation triggers the contraction of the striated muscle fibers of the bulbospongiosus and ischiocavernosus muscles, which are involved in both erection and ejaculation processes. Vasodilation results in the accumulation of blood in the cavernous sinusoids, leading to penile tumescence. Simultaneously, the compression of the emissary veins against the tunica prevents the escape of blood from the cavernosal tissue. The synchronized contraction of striated muscles and increased intracavernosal blood pressure further contribute to the rigidity of the penile erection.

Stages of Penile Erection

Penile erection is a dynamic process that can be divided into distinct phases based on vascular flow, degree of erection, and penile physiology. These phases provide a framework for understanding the different stages of erection [2]:

- Phase 1 (filling phase): Following sexual stimulation, there is an increase in parasympathetic activity, leading to vasodilation. During this phase, blood flow to the cavernous artery increases, resulting in the elongation of the penis.
- Phase 2 (tumescence phase): In this phase, the relaxation of cavernosal smooth muscles allows for maximum blood accumulation in the sinusoidal spaces, leading to penile tumescence and firmness.

- Phase 3 (full erection phase): Once the penile tumescence is achieved, the subtunical veins become compressed against the tunica, preventing the outflow of blood. This results in a full erection, characterized by sustained rigidity.
- Phase 4 (rigid erection phase): The contraction of the bulbospongiosus and ischiocavernosus muscles in this phase leads to an additional increase in intracavernosal pressure. This contributes to a rigid and fully erect penis.
- Phase 5 (detumescence phase): Following sympathetic stimulation, the cavernosal smooth muscles contract, and the venous channels open. This combination reduces intracavernosal pressure, leading to penile softening and detumescence.

Molecular Mechanism of Penile Erection

Physiologically, the stimulation of cavernosal parasympathetic neurons leads to penile erection. This is mediated primarily by the release of a nitric oxide (NO) neurotransmitter in the cavernosal smooth muscle cells. Increased cellular NO leads to the activation of guanylate cyclase and release of a secondary neurotransmitter called cGMP (cyclic guanosine monophosphate). Increased intracellular concentration of cGMP leads to cellular hyperpolarization through phosphatidyl inositol triphosphate–diacyl glycerol–AKT pathway, leading to calcium ion sequestration into the endoplasmic reticulum. Fall in intracellular calcium concentration leads to smooth muscle cellular relaxation. This leads to cavernosal engorgement and subsequent erection [4–6].

Anatomy of the Neurovascular Bundle and Periprostatic Fascia

Periprostatic Nerves

The inferior hypogastric plexus (IHP), also referred to as the pelvic plexus, plays a crucial role in providing innervation to various structures in the pelvic region. Apart from innervating the prostate and seminal vesicles, the pelvic plexus extends visceral branches to other organs, including the bladder, ureter, rectum, membranous urethra, and corpora cavernosa. The IHP is situated in a retroperitoneal position on the lateral surface of the rectum. It typically has a length ranging from 3 to 5.5 cm and a height ranging from 2.5 to 5 cm [7].

The IHP is comprised of sympathetic fibers that originate from the hypogastric nerve. The hypogastric nerve emerges from the anterior horn of the spinal cord and exits through the vertebral foramina spanning from the eleventh thoracic to the second lumbar levels (T11–L2). The IHP is also formed by parasympathetic fibers derive from the pelvic splanchnic nerves, which originate from the anterior rami of S2, S3, and mainly S4 [8]. Costello et al. described three branches from the IHP, namely, superior, anteroinferior, and inferior. The anterior projection courses along the lateral surface of the seminal vesicle and the inferolateral surface of the bladder.

The anteroinferior projection reaches toward the prostatovesical junction and runs obliquely along the lateral surface of the prostate. Lastly, the inferior projection travels between the rectum and the posterolateral surface of the prostate, forming the neurovascular bundle (NVB) [9].

The nerve-sparing prostatectomy was first described by Walsh and Donker in 1982. In their original description, they reported the presence of a single neurovascular bundle (NVB) on each side of the prostate at its posterolateral surface [10]. However, subsequent histopathological studies have revealed a more intricate distribution of the periprostatic nerves. For instance, Tewari et al. identified a "neural hammock-like distribution" characterized by three primary zones: the proximal neural plate (PNP) or pelvic plexus, the predominant neurovascular bundle (PNB), and the accessory neural pathways (ANP) (Figs. 1.2 and 1.3) [7, 11, 12]. Similarly, Takenaka et al. described a spray-like arrangement of the periprostatic nerves [13].

Sievert et al. conducted a study using serial whole-mounted sections stained for different types of nerves (sympathetic, parasympathetic, and sensory). They found that parasympathetic nerves exhibited distinct patterns depending on the prostate region. At the base, these nerves were primarily distributed in an anterolateral fashion. In the midsection, a posterolateral distribution was prominent, while at the apex, the distribution shifted toward a posterolateral to posterior pattern. This research highlights the intricate regional variations in the distribution of parasympathetic nerves within the prostate [14]. Panebianco et al. conducted a study using three-dimensional models and the diffusion tensor imaging technique (DTI) to examine the distribution pattern of periprostatic nerves. Their findings also revealed interesting variations across different regions of the prostate. For instance, a greater concentration of nerve fibers was observed in the

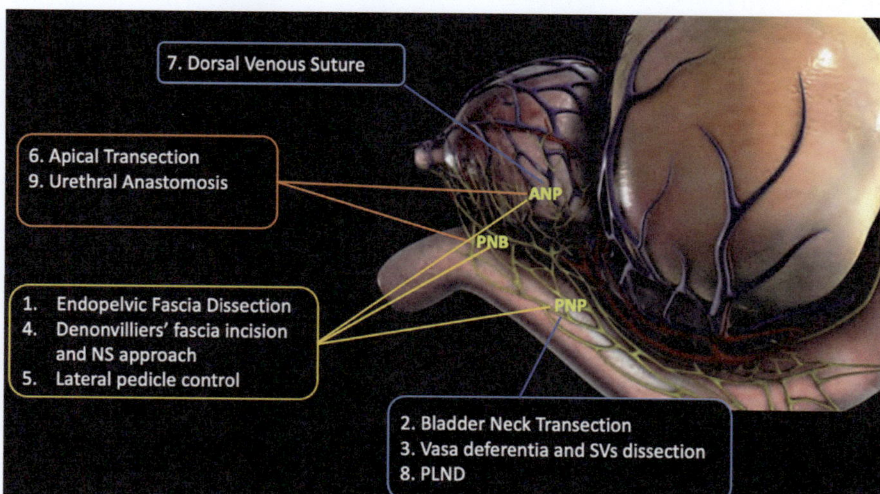

Fig. 1.2 Critical steps during RARP where potential injury to the neural hammock may occur. (Reproduced with permission from Pedraza et al. [12])

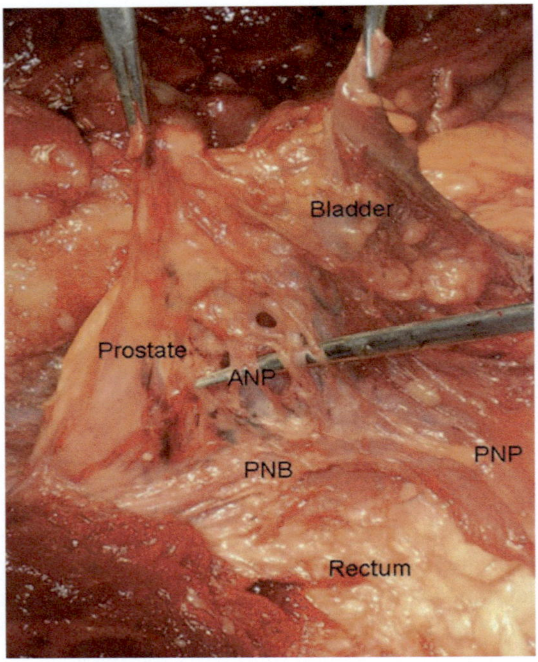

Fig. 1.3 Lateral view of PNP, PNB, and ANP. Fresh cadaver dissection showing that the neural pathway from the PNP is a spray-like distribution. The prostate and bladder are lifted up by the forceps. (Reproduced with permission from Tewari et al. [7])

posterolateral area at the base of the prostate. Within the midgland of the prostate, around two-thirds of the nerve fibers were concentrated in the posterolateral area. Conversely, at the prostatic apex, there were no differences in the distribution between the posterolateral and anterolateral areas [15]. These findings highlight the complex distribution and varied nature of the nerve network surrounding the prostate.

Periprostatic Fascia

The prostate is enveloped by three distinct fascial structures: Denonvilliers' fascia, the prostatic fascia, and the endopelvic fascia. Denonvilliers' fascia is situated at the posterior aspect, closely adhering to the prostate and creating a separation between the prostate and the rectum. Additionally, it covers the posterior surface of the seminal vesicles. The prostatic fascia surrounds the prostate gland and exhibits direct continuity with the fibromuscular stroma in the anterior and anterolateral regions. Laterally, it merges with the endopelvic fascia, while posteriorly, it seamlessly blends with Denonvilliers' fascia [16]. The prostatic fascia is often composed of multiple layers that extend over the prostate, incorporating both collagenous and adipose tissues [17].

Physiology of Urinary Continence and Anatomy of the Urinary Sphincter and Hood

The Urethral Sphincter Complex

The urethral sphincter complex plays an important role in continence preservation. Anatomically, it can be subdivided into two different entities: the internal urethral sphincter (IUS) and the external urethral sphincter (EUS). The former is composed of smooth muscle that is continuous with the detrusor muscle of the bladder. It is located at the junction of the bladder neck and proximal urethra, which in males is demarcated by the prostatic base (Fig. 1.4). The IUS forms a "horseshoe"-like structure that is controlled by the autonomic nervous system. During voiding, the IUS relaxes via parasympathetic input. At rest, sympathetic input prevails and prevents the continuous egress of urine through tonic contraction of the sphincter [18].

The EUS conversely is composed primarily of outer striated skeletal muscle fibers (rhabdosphincter) and inner smooth muscle fibers (lissosphincter). It has been long believed to be under voluntary control. Its role lies in mediating the coaptation of the urethra. Therefore, malfunction of the EUS can lead to urinary incontinence. In men, the EUS is formed by circular muscle fibers within the membranous segment of the urethra and is classically defined as having an "omega" shape [18].

Though traditionally the EUS has been believed to be under somatic innervation via the pudendal nerves (which in turn are formed by the S2–S4 nerve roots), recent evidence would suggest that there exists a component of autonomic innervation as well [19]. In fact, Nyangoh Timoh et al. have shown that autonomic nerves originating from the inferior hypogastric plexus (IHP) run along the posteromedial aspect of the prostatic apex and penetrate through the rectourethral muscle on their way to the EUS. The authors also demonstrate that autonomic nerves running within the neurovascular bundles along the posterolateral edge of the prostate also innervate the EUS. The act of micturition is predicated on sequential parasympathetic input to the IUS (leading to its relaxation) and voluntary (or somatic) relaxation of the EUS [20].

The "Hood" Complex and Its Relevance During Radical Prostatectomy

The key structures that provide support include the pubovesical/puboprostatic ligaments (PV/PPLs), endopelvic fascia, fascial tendinous arch of the pelvis, levator ani muscles, and Denonvilliers' fascia [21]. The supportive mechanism plays a crucial role in keeping the bladder, prostate, and external sphincter in their proper positions

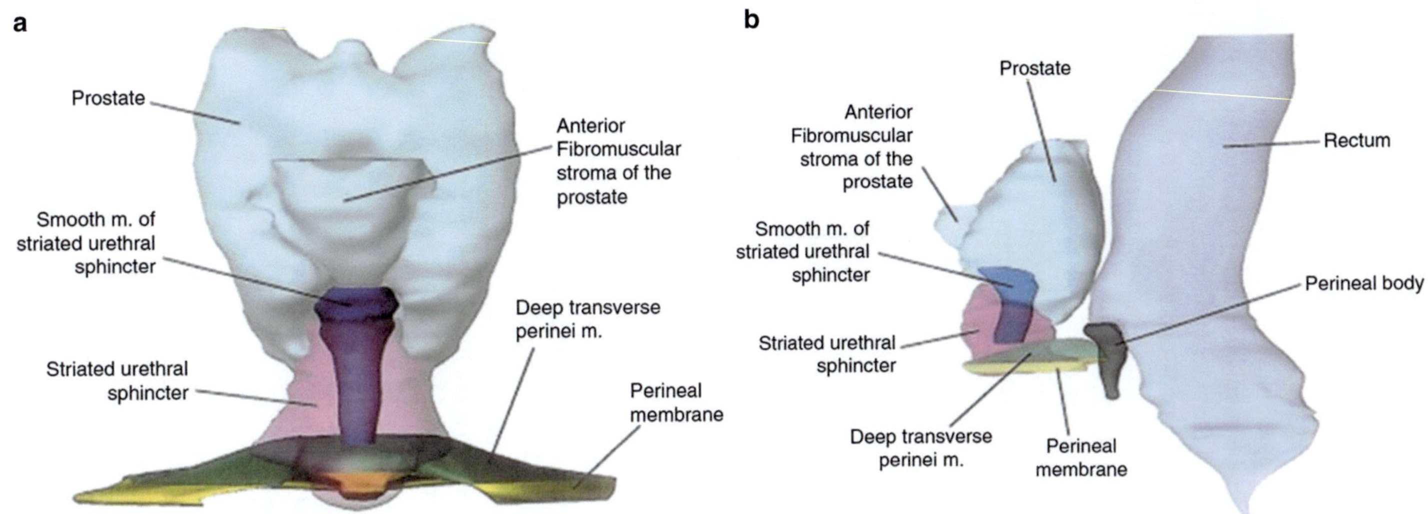

Fig. 1.4 Structure of the male striated urethral sphincter. (**a**) Anterior projection shows the cone shape of the sphincter and the smooth muscle of the sphincter. (**b**) Viewed laterally, the anterior wall of the sphincter is nearly twice the length of the posterior wall, although both are of comparable thickness. (Reproduced from Chung et al. [26], with permission from Elsevier)

within the pelvic cavity. When intra-abdominal pressure increases, these structures prevent the descent of the sphincteric mechanisms (urethral hypermobility) and maintain the angulation of the vesico-prostatic junction. The PV/PPLs are paired extensions of the fibrocollagenous tissue that originate from the lower front surface of the prostate and the front surface of the urethral sphincter. They extend to the periosteum over the back lower surface of the pubis bone. These ligaments play a role in supporting the bladder, prostate, and external sphincter, effectively suspending the internal and external sphincter within the pelvic cavity [22].

The endopelvic fascia consists of two layers (parietal and visceral) that, along with the fascial tendinous arch of pelvis, form a continuous framework. This framework extends from the PV/PPLs to the ischial spine. It provides additional support to the pelvic structures. The levator ani muscle forms the floor of the pelvic cavity. It is composed of fibers from the pubococcygeus muscle at the front and the iliococcygeus muscle at the back. Near the urogenital hiatus, the fibers of the levator ani muscle thicken to flank the junction between the prostate and urethra. This thickened portion is known as puboperinealis. It extends from the pubis bone at the front to the perineal body at the back. When the puboperinealis muscle contracts, it pulls the urethra upward and forward toward the pubis bone. Simultaneously, the rhabdosphincter contracts and pulls the urethra downward and backward toward the perineal body, with the posterior musculofascial plate acting as the fulcrum. This double-sling mechanism helps in closing the urethra and maintaining continence (Fig. 1.5) [21, 23].

Urinary incontinence and sexual dysfunction following radical prostatectomy mediate postsurgical quality of life. As such, an abundance of literature exists attempting to determine ways by which to mitigate these consequences while optimally preserving cancer control. The “hood” technique represents an anterior surgical approach to performing a radical prostatectomy that preserves structures within the space of Retzius that mediate urinary continence. These structures include the detrusor apron, the arcus tendineus, the puboprostatic ligaments, and the anterior vessels. Following a circumferential apical dissection and control of the dorsal venous complex, development of the “hood” proceeds. This involves creation of a plane between the anterior fibromuscular stroma of the prostate and the muscular fibers of the detrusor apron. Eventually, once the urethrovesical anastomosis has been performed, the arcus tendineus is sutured to the detrusor apron, thereby allowing for stabilization of the urethrovesical junction. As Wagaskar et al. have shown, the “hood” technique has key benefits: early return to continence and a low rate of positive surgical margins [24].

Take-Home Message

The foundation of any surgery is intimate understanding of anatomy and structural relations. In order to effectively incorporate surgical techniques to optimize urinary continence and erectile function, it is crucial for the surgeon to prospectively identify the neurovascular hammock, the subtle change in muscle fiber directions when performing a precise bladder neck dissection, and the difference in prostatic urethra and membranous urethra location for urethral length preservation. The surgeon can

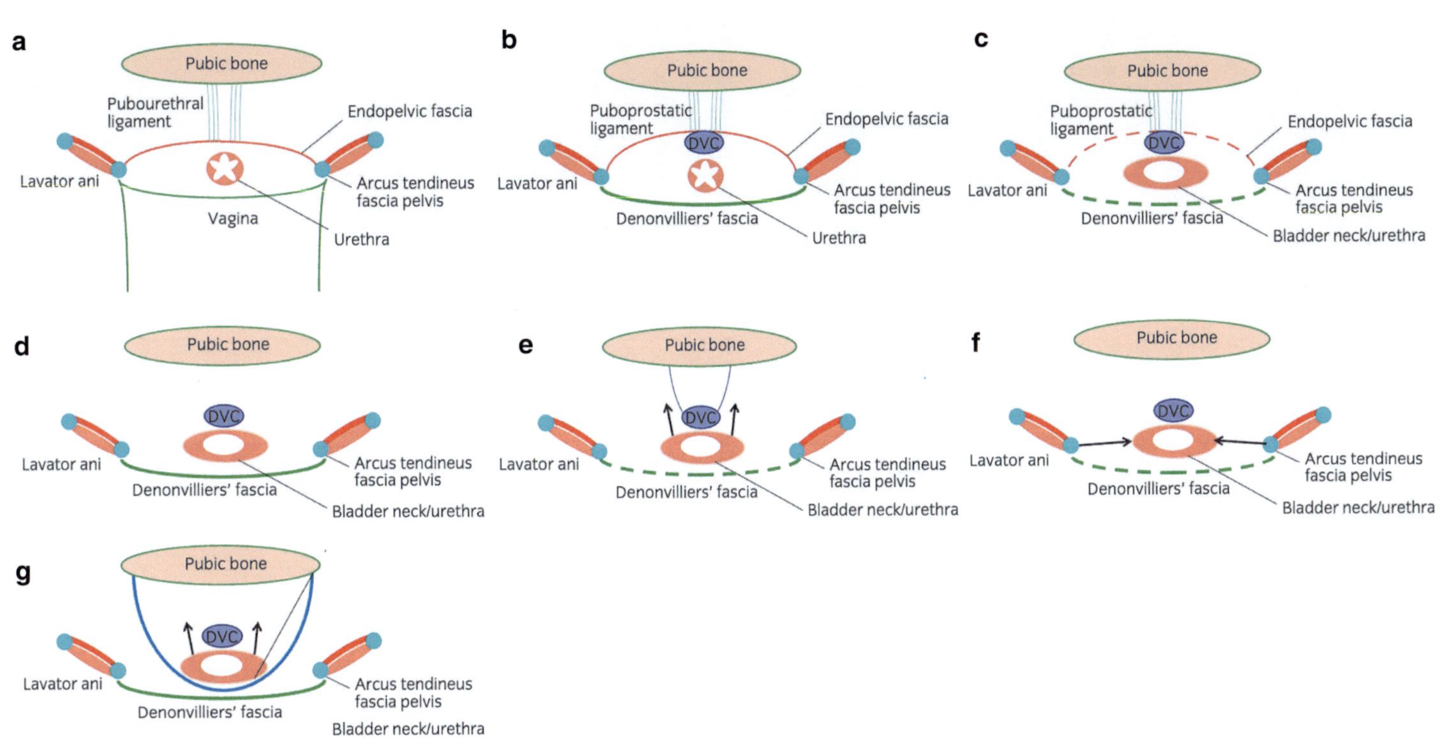

Fig. 1.5 Supporting system in the pelvis and reconstruction and reinforcement during RARP. (**a**) Structural support in the female pelvis. (**b**) Structural support in the male pelvis. (**c**) Structural changes after radical prostatectomy. (**d**) Posterior reconstruction of the rhabdosphincter. (**e**) Anterior retropubic suspension. (**f**) Reattachment of the arcus tendineus to the bladder neck. (**g**) Bone-anchored bladder neck sling suspension. DVC dorsal vein complex. (Reproduced from Kojima et al. [27], with permission from Wiley)

also utilize the anatomy of the pelvic floor to reconstruct suspensory support of the bladder and urethra after prostatectomy. These specific techniques will be further discussed in subsequent chapters.

References

1. Weech D, Ameer MA, Ashurst JV. Anatomy, Abdomen and Pelvis, Penis Dorsal Nerve. [Updated 2023 Aug 8]. In: StatPearls [Internet]. Treasure Island (FL): StatPearls Publishing; 2024. Available from: https://www.ncbi.nlm.nih.gov/books/NBK525966/.
2. Dean RC, Lue TF. Physiology of penile erection and pathophysiology of erectile dysfunction. Urol Clin North Am. 2005;32(4):379.
3. Anderson KE, Wagner G. Physiology of penile erection. Physiol Rev. 1995;75(1):191–236. https://doi.org/10.1152/physrev.1995.75.1.191.
4. Sangiorgi G, Cereda A, Benedetto D, et al. Clinical management of erectile dysfunction in patients affected by coronary artery disease: a review. Biomedicine. 2021;9(4):432.
5. Lue TF. Erectile dysfunction. NEJM. 2000;342(24):1802–13.
6. Walsh MP. The Ayerst Award Lecture 1990 / La Confkrence Ayerst 1990. Calcium-dependent mechanisms of regulation of smooth muscle contraction. Biochem Cell Biol. 1991;69(12):771–800.
7. Tewari A, Takenaka A, Mtui E, et al. The proximal neurovascular plate and the tri-zonal neural architecture around the prostate gland: importance in the athermal robotic technique of nerve-sparing prostatectomy. BJU Int. 2006;98(2):314–23. https://doi.org/10.1111/j.1464-410X.2006.06266.x.
8. Mauroy B, Demondion X, Drizenko A, et al. The inferior hypogastric plexus (pelvic plexus): its importance in neural preservation techniques. Surg Radiol Anat. 2003;25(1):6–15. https://doi.org/10.1007/s00276-002-0083-9.
9. Costello AJ, Brooks M, Cole OJ. Anatomical studies of the neurovascular bundle and cavernosal nerves. BJU Int. 2004;94(7):1071–6. https://doi.org/10.1111/j.1464-410X.2004.05106.x.
10. Walsh PC, Donker PJ. Impotence following radical prostatectomy: insight into etiology and prevention. J Urol. 1982;128(3):492–7. https://doi.org/10.1016/S0022-5347(17)53012-8.
11. Tewari AK, Srivastava A, Huang MW, et al. Anatomical grades of nerve sparing: a risk-stratified approach to neural-hammock sparing during robot-assisted radical prostatectomy (RARP). BJU Int. 2011;108(6 B):984–92. https://doi.org/10.1111/j.1464-410X.2011.10565.x.
12. Pedraza AM, Pandav K, Menon M, et al. Current strategies to improve erectile function in patients undergoing radical prostatectomy-intraoperative scenario. Urol Oncol Semin Orig Investig. 2022;40(3):79–86. https://doi.org/10.1016/j.urolonc.2021.12.003.
13. Takenaka A, Murakami G, Soga H, Han SH, Arai Y, Fujisawa M. Anatomical analysis of the neurovascular bundle supplying penile cavernous tissue to ensure a reliable nerve graft after radical prostatectomy. J Urol. 2004;172(3):1032–5. https://doi.org/10.1097/01.ju.0000135648.33110.df.
14. Sievert KD, Hennenlotter J, Dillenburg T, et al. Extended periprostatic nerve distributions on the prostate surface confirmed using diffusion tensor imaging. BJU Int. 2019;123(6):995–1004. https://doi.org/10.1111/bju.14508.
15. Panebianco V, Barchetti F, Sciarra A, et al. In vivo 3D neuroanatomical evaluation of periprostatic nerve plexus with 3T-MR diffusion tensor imaging. Eur J Radiol. 2013;82(10):1677–82. https://doi.org/10.1016/j.ejrad.2013.05.013.
16. Raychaudhuri B, Cahill D. Pelvic fasciae in urology. Ann R Coll Surg Engl. 2008;90(8):633–7. https://doi.org/10.1308/003588408X321611.

17. Kiyoshima K, Yokomizo A, Yoshida T, et al. Anatomical features of periprostatic tissue and its surroundings: a histological analysis of 79 radical retropubic prostatectomy specimens. Jpn J Clin Oncol. 2004;34(8):463–8. https://doi.org/10.1093/jjco/hyh078.
18. Jung J, Ahn HK, Huh Y. Clinical and functional anatomy of the urethral sphincter. Int Neurourol J. 2012;16(3):102–6. https://doi.org/10.5213/inj.2012.16.3.102.
19. Bessede T, Sooriakumaran P, Takenaka A, Tewari A. Neural supply of the male urethral sphincter: comprehensive anatomical review and implications for continence recovery after radical prostatectomy. World J Urol. 2017;35(4):549–65. https://doi.org/10.1007/s00345-016-1901-8.
20. Nyangoh Timoh K, Moszkowicz D, Creze M, et al. The male external urethral sphincter is autonomically innervated. Clin Anat. 2021;34(2):263–71. https://doi.org/10.1002/ca.23698.
21. Walz J, Epstein JI, Ganzer R, Graefen M, Guazzoni G, Kaouk J, Menon M, Mottrie A, Myers RP, Patel V, Tewari A, Villers A, Artibani W. A Critical Analysis of the Current Knowledge of Surgical Anatomy of the Prostate Related to Optimisation of Cancer Control and Preservation of Continence and Erection in Candidates for Radical Prostatectomy: An Update. Eur Urol. 2016;70(2):301–11. https://doi.org/10.1016/j.eururo.2016.01.026. Epub 2016. PMID: 26850969.
22. Brooks JD, Chao WM, Kerr J. Male pelvic anatomy reconstructed from the visible human data set. J Urol. 1998;159(3):868–72. https://doi.org/10.1016/S0022-5347(01)63757-1.
23. Myers RP, Cahill DR, Kay PA, et al. Puboperineales: muscular boundaries of the male urogenital hiatus in 3D from magnetic resonance imaging. J Urol. 2000;164(4):1412–5. https://doi.org/10.1016/S0022-5347(05)67208-4.
24. Wagaskar VG, Mittal A, Sobotka S, et al. Hood technique for robotic radical prostatectomy—preserving periurethral anatomical structures in the space of retzius and sparing the pouch of douglas, enabling early return of continence without compromising surgical margin rates. Eur Urol. 2021;80(2):213–21. https://doi.org/10.1016/j.eururo.2020.09.044.
25. Greg T MacLennan Hinman's atlas of uro-surgical anatomy, 2nd ed, Saunders an imprint of Elsevier, Philadelphia.
26. Chung B, Sommer G, Brooks JD. Surgical, radiographic and endoscopic anatomy of the male pelvis. In: Wein A, Kavoussi L, Partin W, Peters C, editors. Campbell-Walsh urology. Philadelphia: Elsevier; 2016. p. 1611–30.
27. Kojima Y, Takahashi N, Haga N, Nomiya M, Yanagida T, Ishibashi K, et al. Urinary incontinence after robot-assisted radical prostatectomy: pathophysiology and intraoperative techniques to improve surgical outcome. Int J Urol. 2013;20(11):1052–63.

Imaging Modalities for Prostate Cancer

2

Hala Khasawneh, Dina Hamdan,
and Pamela Causa Andrieu

Abbreviations

ADC	Apparent diffusion coefficient
AUC	Area under the curve
DCE	Dynamic contrast-enhanced
FACBC	Anti-1-amino-3-^{18}F-fluorocyclobutane-1–carboxylic acid
FDG	Fluorodeoxyglucose
MRI	Magnetic resonance imaging
NCCN	National Comprehensive Cancer Network
PI-RADS	Prostate Imaging Reporting and Data System
PSA	Prostate-specific antigen
PSMA	Prostate-specific membrane antigen
RECIST	Response Evaluation Criteria in Solid Tumors
TRUS	Transrectal ultrasound

The original version of the chapter has been revised. A correction to this chapter can be found at https://doi.org/10.1007/978-3-031-64245-6_14

H. Khasawneh
Department of Radiology – University of Texas Southwestern Medical Center, Dallas, TX, USA

D. Hamdan
Department of Radiology – Ichan School of Medicine at Mount Sinai, New York, NY, USA

P. Causa Andrieu (✉)
Department of Radiology – Mayo Clinic, Rochester, MN, USA

S. Razdan, S. Razdan (eds.), *Urinary Continence and Sexual Function After Robotic Prostatectomy, Radiation, and Novel Therapies*,
https://doi.org/10.1007/978-3-031-64245-6_2

Introduction

Imaging plays a vital role as a noninvasive tool in the management of patients with prostate cancer, including in diagnosis, staging, and posttreatment follow-up. Moreover, advances both in the imaging and treatment of prostate cancer have ushered a paradigm shift in prostate cancer management, offering opportunities for early detection, improved locoregional staging, and the selection of patients to active surveillance versus radical treatment. Multiple imaging modalities are available depending on the clinical indication and institutional availability and preference. This chapter will discuss the role of commonly used imaging modalities in several common clinical scenarios. Moreover, radiomics and artificial intelligence applications will be discussed toward the end of the chapter.

Imaging Modalities

Magnetic Resonance Imaging

Magnetic resonance imaging (MRI) is currently the primary modality used in the imaging assessment of patients with prostate cancer. MRI offers superior anatomic delineation of the prostate and of its zonal anatomy as well as superior visualization of adjacent pelvic structures. Typically, MRI is performed using a 1.5 or 3 Tesla unit with a multichannel pelvic phased-array receiver coil and optionally an endorectal coil [1].

Multiparametric MRI combines the anatomical sequences of T1-weighted imaging (T1WI) and multiplanar T2-weighted imaging (T2WI) with the functional sequences of dynamic contrast-enhanced (DCE) imaging and diffusion-weighted imaging (DWI) with apparent diffusion coefficient (ADC) mapping. Meanwhile, biparametric MRI combines only T2WI and DWI. The clinical indications for multiparametric and biparametric MRI are summarized in Table 2.1. T1WI with a wide field of view offers superior soft tissue resolution to differentiate the prostate from periprostatic fat and to detect osseous lesions in the pelvis. T2WI is used to depict the zonal anatomy of the prostate (the peripheral, transition, and central zones) and to detect signal abnormalities indicative of various prostate pathologies, including but not limited to cancer,

Table 2.1 Clinical indications of bi- and multiparametric MRI according to PI-RADS V2

Biparametric MRI	Multiparametric MRI (with intravenous contrast)
Treatment naïve	Prior hormonal therapy
	Prior radiotherapy
	Prior local therapy
	Prior radical prostatectomy
	Limited DWI, e.g., in the presence of bilateral hip prosthesis

prostatitis, and normal variants. Functional sequences increase the sensitivity and positive predictive value in detecting and diagnosing prostate cancer.

Prostate Anatomy on MRI

The prostate is divided into the apex, the mid-gland, and the base. The apex constitutes the lower-third of the prostate, the base the upper-third, and the mid-gland the middle-third. The mid-gland includes the verumontanum, which is a longitudinal mucosal fold forming an elliptical segment of the mid-prostatic urethra at the point where the ejaculatory ducts enter the urethra [2].

The zonal anatomy of the prostate is well delineated on MRI, with each zone characterized by distinct signal characteristics (Fig. 2.1). The prostate is composed

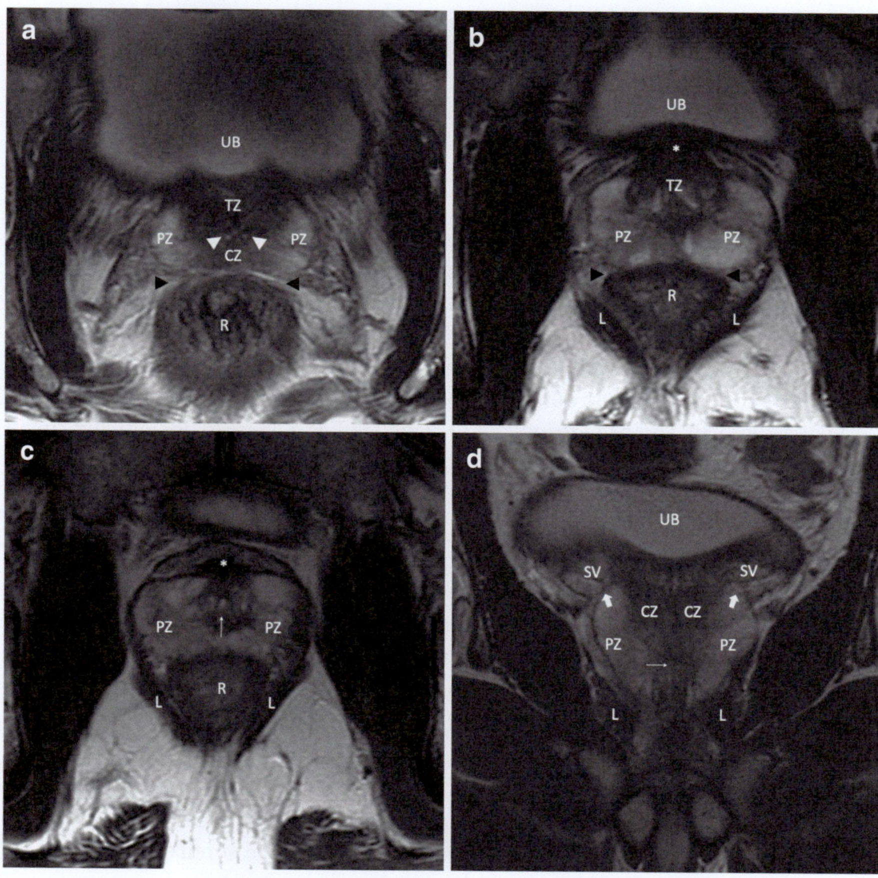

Fig. 2.1 Normal zonal anatomy. Prostate MRI in a 40-year-old patient. Axial T2WI at the level of the base (**a**), mid-gland (**b**), and apex (**c**). Coronal T2WI (**d**). PZ, peripheral zone; CZ, central zone; TZ, transition zone; R, rectum; UB, urinary bladder; L, levator ani; asterisk, anterior fibromuscular stroma; white arrow, distal prostatic urethra; white arrowheads, ejaculatory ducts; black arrowheads, rectoprostatic angle; SV, seminal vesicles; block arrows, prostate–seminal vesicle angle. Note T2 hypointense linear bands in the bilateral peripheral zone are non-specific and probably represent inflammatory changes

of three distinct zones with different embryologic origins: the peripheral zone, central zone, and transition zone. The cup-shaped peripheral zone extends from the base to the apex, surrounds the distal prostatic urethra, and is separated from the central and transition zones by a fibrous layer. The peripheral zone is deficient anteriorly, where it is replaced by the anterior fibromuscular stroma [3]. The peripheral zone has high signal intensity on T2WI due to its abundant ductal and acinar elements. Meanwhile, the cone-shaped central zone is located at the base between the peripheral and transition zones, surrounds the ejaculatory ducts, and narrows to an apex at the verumontanum. In contrast to the peripheral zone, the central zone has homogeneous low T2WI signal intensity. Another zone, the transition zone, extends from the base to the apex and is predominantly anterolateral to the prostatic urethra. The transition zone consists of two small lobules of glandular tissue surrounding the proximal prostatic urethra. On MRI, the transition zone usually appears as nodular areas of varying signal intensity, depending on the relative amount of glandular and stromal hyperplasia [4]; hyperplasia of the glandular elements results in higher T2WI signal intensity, whereas stromal hyperplasia results in lower T2WI signal intensity.

The seminal vesicles are paired grapelike pouches filled with high T2WI signal intensity fluid located caudolaterally to the prostate gland. Neurovascular bundles travel posterolaterally on both sides and give off branches into the prostate at the apex and base [5].

The anterior fibromuscular stroma forms the convexity of the anterior external surface. It lacks glandular tissue and thus demonstrates low T2WI signal intensity. Superiorly, it is continuous with the detrusor muscle. The apical half blends into the gland and the muscle of the pelvic diaphragm. It thins laterally and posteriorly to form a fibrous "capsule" surrounding the prostate gland (of note, the prostate lacks a true capsule) [5]. The pseudocapsule is visualized as a sharply demarcated rim at the posterolateral aspects of the prostate on T2WI.

Role of MRI in Primary Staging

MRI has a high detection rate when it comes to lesions with a volume of 0.5 cm^3 or greater [6]. On MRI, prostate cancer appears as a nodule with low T2WI signal intensity, diffusion restriction, and early enhancement and washout. Conversely, linear and wedge-shaped low T2WI signal abnormalities are often due to inflammatory changes and are less likely to be prostate cancer. DWI is valuable for detecting prostate cancer in the peripheral zone but not in the transition zone as benign prostate hyperplasia nodules in the transition zone may have restricted diffusion and present a pitfall. For detecting prostate cancer in the transition zone, T2WI is the guiding sequence, whereby prostate cancer in the transition zone will show a distinctive appearance with irregular indistinct margins, often referred to as the "erased charcoal" sign (Fig. 2.2) [7, 8].

MRI has gained importance in the management of patients with prostate cancer as it improves local staging by identifying the presence of extraprostatic extension and seminal vesicle invasion. Signs that indicate the presence of extraprostatic extension include increased capsular contact, capsular bulge and irregularity, obliteration of the rectoprostatic angle, and asymmetry of the neurovascular bundles (Fig. 2.3) [8]. MRI

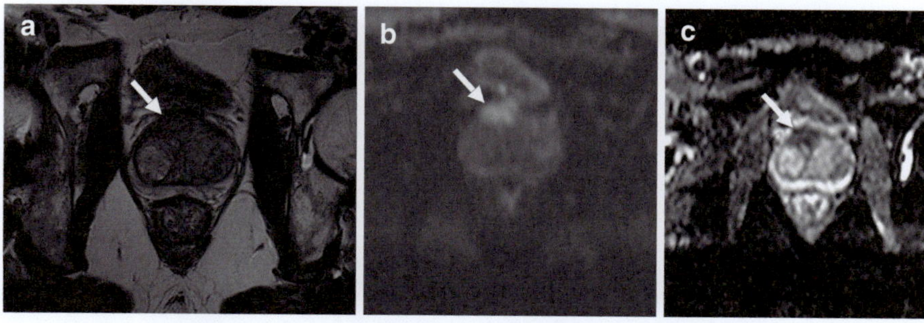

Fig. 2.2 Transition zone tumor. Prostate MRI in a 70-year-old patient with elevated PSA. T2WI (**a**) shows a non-circumscribed hypointense lesion (arrow) with indistinct margin “erased charcoal” in the anterior transition zone involving the anterior fibromuscular stroma. Corresponding hyperintense signal on DWI (**b**) and hypointense signal on ADC (**c**) is seen

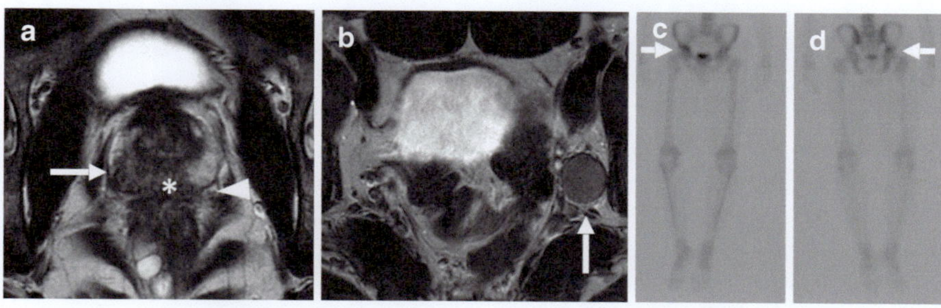

Fig. 2.3 Tumor with extracapsular extension and bone metastasis. Prostate MRI in a 36-year-old patient with elevated PSA. Axial T2WI (**a**) shows a large tumor (arrow) involving the posterior aspect of the right peripheral zone and crossing the midline posteriorly (asterisk). The tumor extends beyond the capsule posteriorly (white arrowhead). Axial T2WI at a more superior level (**b**) shows an enlarged and rounded left obturator suspected nodal metastasis (arrow). Technetium-99 m MDP bone scan anterior view (**c**) and posterior view (**d**) show uptake in the right acetabulum (arrow), suspicious for osseous metastasis

has a relatively high pooled specificity of 87% but a modest sensitivity of 55% for detecting extraprostatic extension [9]. A grading system has been developed to assess the risk of extraprostatic extension. Grade 1, with a risk of 24%, is assigned to cases with either a curvilinear contact length of 1.5 cm or capsular bulge and irregularity. Grade 2, with a risk of 38%, corresponds to the presence of both curvilinear contact length and capsular budge and irregularity. Finally, grade 3, with a risk of 66%, corresponds to the presence of a frank capsular breach or invasion of adjacent structures [10]. Meanwhile, signs that indicate seminal vesicle invasion include replacement of the normal bright/high T2WI signal intensity of the seminal vesicles with homogeneous low signal, loss of known tubular appearance of the seminal vesicles, and diffusion restriction (Fig. 2.4). Besides identifying the presence of extraprostatic extension and seminal vesicle invasion, MRI is also useful for identifying invasion of adjacent pelvic structures including the rectum, bladder, external urethral sphincter, pelvic side walls, and pelvic floor muscles.

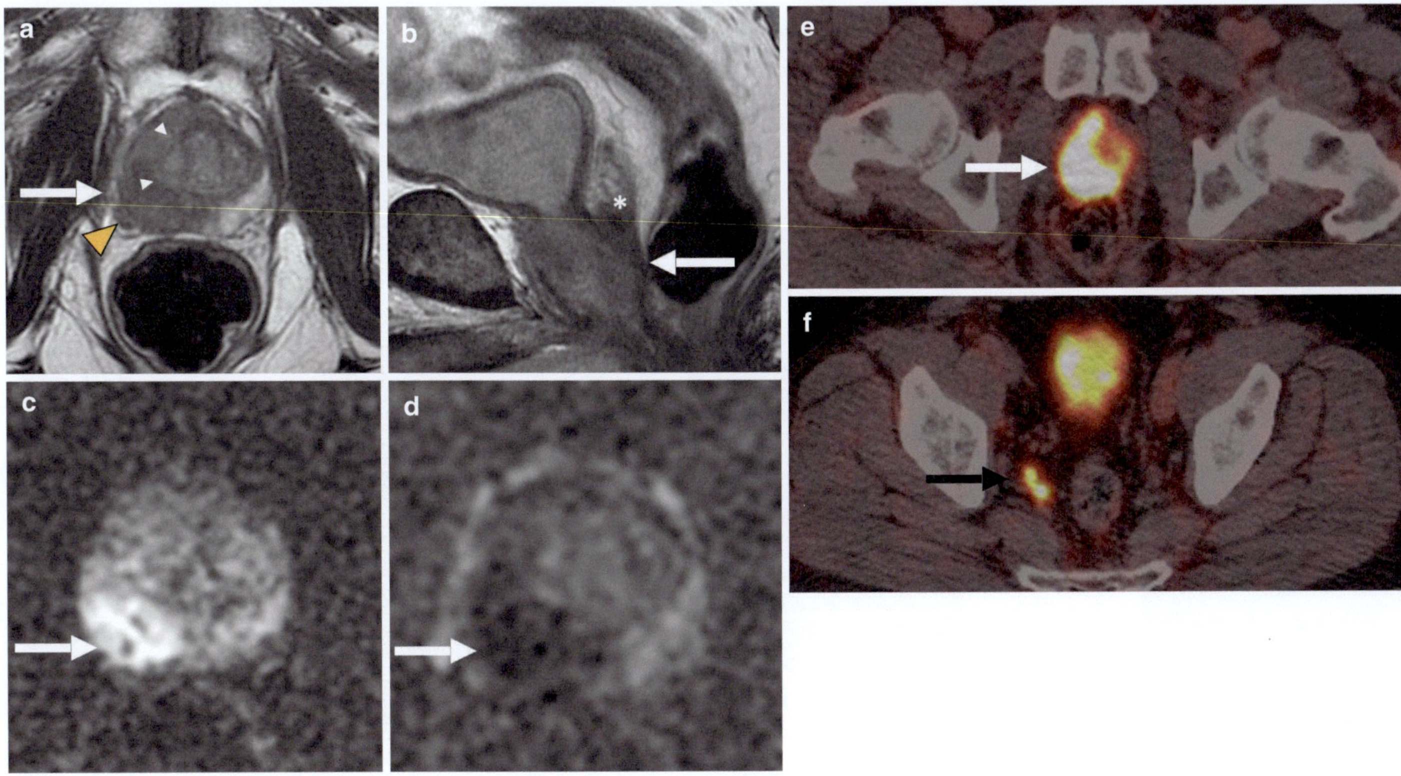

Fig. 2.4 Tumor with extracapsular extension and seminal vesicle invasion. Prostate MRI in a 64-year-old patient with elevated PSA. Axial T2WI (**a**) and sagittal T2WI (**b**) show a large tumor (arrow) involving the anterior and posterior aspects of the right peripheral zone from the apex to the base. There is probable involvement of the transition zone (white arrowhead), extension beyond the capsule posterolaterally (yellow arrowhead), and invasion of the inferior tip of the right seminal vesicle (*). Axial DWI (**c**) shows high signal intensity in the lesion (arrow) with a corresponding low signal intensity on ADC (**d**). Gallium-68 PSMA PET/CT (**e, f**) reveals hypermetabolic prostatic tumor (white arrow) and metastatic lymph node (black arrow)

Lesions in the prostate are evaluated and categorized based on a five-point scale reflecting the likelihood of clinically significant prostate cancer, according to the American College of Radiology Prostate Imaging Reporting and Data System (PI-RADS) [1]. PI-RADS, the most recent version being version 2.1, was established to provide guidelines regarding the minimum acceptable technical parameters for imaging acquisition and to offer a reproducible prostate MRI reporting system with the intended result of improving the prediction of clinically significant prostate cancer. According to the level of suspicion of clinically significant prostate cancer, patients can be assigned to active surveillance or radical treatments such as radiation and surgery [1, 11].

Role of MRI in Detecting Metastases

Whole-body MRI has the advantage of being a one-stop shop for primary tumor assessment, disease staging, and treatment planning. Currently, it is one of the most used imaging tools for detecting metastases, particularly bone metastases (Fig. 2.5). Whole-body MRI involves obtaining multiple consecutive high spatial resolution anatomic and functional sequences for the whole body, which are subsequently reconstructed and fused [12]. The sequences are constantly updated to optimize metastasis detection and mainly include T2WI, T1WI, and DWI, with the acquisition of fat-suppressed images or Short-TI Inversion Recovery images [12].

The introduction of the METastasis Reporting and Data System for Prostate Cancer (MET-RADS-P), a standardized protocol guideline for optimal acquisition, interpretation, and reporting of whole-body MRI, is promising [13, 14]. However, further studies are required to evaluate and validate the impact of MET-RADS-P in clinical practice [14].

Role of MRI in Treatment Planning

In terms of treatment planning, organ-confined prostate cancer with a low risk of extraprostatic extension allows the patient the opportunity for nerve-preserving radical prostatectomy, which reduces postoperative complications such as erectile dysfunction and urinary incontinence. Needless to say, nerve-preserving radical prostatectomy must be done accurately as potential positive margins can introduce the risk of recurrence, and MRI is especially useful for treatment planning in this setting. MRI can also be used to guide radiation treatment and focal ablative therapies, particularly in terms of patient selection, treatment planning, and intraprocedural monitoring, although its use as such is mainly still limited to clinical trial settings. MRI can also assist in determining several important factors such as the bilaterality, localization, size, and extent of the lesion to determine patient eligibility and whether to perform partial versus total gland ablation.

MRI-Guided Biopsy

A meta-analysis reported that MRI-guided biopsy has 50% higher detection rates of prostate cancer compared with standard transrectal ultrasound (TRUS)-guided biopsy, with higher detection rates particularly of carcinoma in situ [15]. In addition, MRI-guided biopsy has shown high negative predictive values of up to 92%

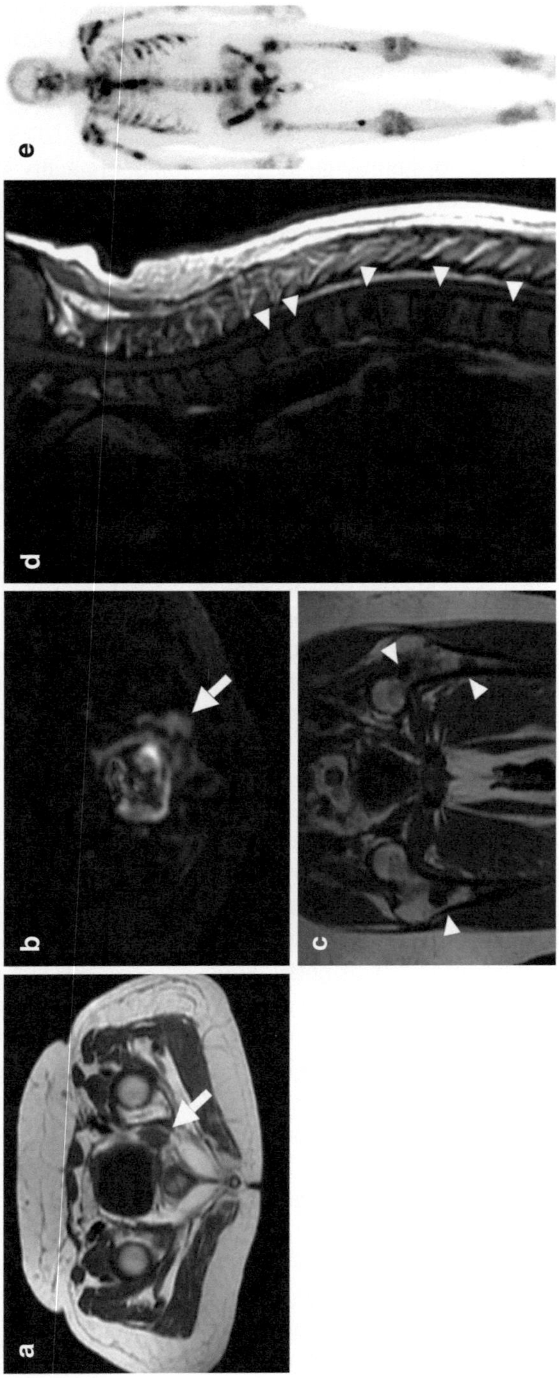

Fig. 2.5 Recurrent tumor and bone metastases. Whole-body MRI in a 51-year-old patient who underwent prostatectomy for Gleason 4 + 5 tumor. Axial T1WI of the pelvis (**a**) shows a hypointense lesion (arrow) in the left pelvic sidewall with diffusion restriction (**b**) consistent with local tumor recurrence. Coronal T1WI of the pelvis (**c**) and sagittal T1WI of the cervicodorsal spine (**d**) shows widespread osseus metastases (arrowheads). Technetium-99 m MDP bone scan anterior view (**e**) shows widespread uptake in the axial and appendicular skeleton consistent with osseous metastases

and a sensitivity value of up to 93% [16]. Of note, MRI-guided biopsy can be done as part of MRI/TRUS fusion biopsy or simply as in-bore MRI-guided biopsy [16].

Of note, two leading prospective studies, PROMIS and PRECISION, provided evidence supporting the superiority of MRI-guided biopsy for prostate cancer detection and for the minimization of overtreatment of patients with low-volume and low-grade disease which is associated with adverse cancer-related events [15, 17]. PROMIS, a multicenter prospective study, confirmed the superiority of MRI-guided biopsy compared with TRUS-guided biopsy, whereby MRI-guided biopsy had a significantly higher sensitivity and higher negative predictive value compared with TRUS. As such, MRI-guided biopsy helped to spare up to one-quarter of patients from undergoing invasive biopsy. For clinically significant prostate cancer, MRI-guided biopsy was found to be more sensitive but less specific (93% and 41%, respectively) compared with TRUS-guided biopsy (48% and 96%, respectively) [18]. The PRECISION study confirmed that MRI-stratified pathways, by using either MRI-guided biopsy alone or in conjunction with TRUS-guided biopsy, can increase the detection rate of clinically significant prostate cancer up to 1.45 times compared with TRUS-guided biopsy alone in biopsy-naïve patients [15, 17].

Role of MRI in Active Surveillance

Active surveillance is a widely accepted strategy targeting low-risk prostate cancer patients. Patients undergoing active surveillance are monitored and do not undergo treatment until there is clinical or radiological progression. This primarily aims to avoid unwarranted treatment side effects, whether from surgery, radiation, or ablation therapy, in clinically indolent cancers. Among other guidelines, the National Comprehensive Cancer Network (NCCN) criteria for very-low-risk prostate cancer are those with clinical stage $\leq$ T1c, Gleason score $\leq$ 6, <3/12 benign cores on biopsy, <50% cancer-positive tissue in each biopsy core, prostate-specific antigen (PSA) <10 ng/mL, and life expectancy >20 years [19, 20].

Prostate cancer progression is detected by increasing PSA > 10 ng/mL and a Gleason score of $\geq$7 at repeat biopsy. Currently, imaging progression on MRI is not included as a criterion for progression during active surveillance, and the determination of progression is based solely on clinical and pathological information. However, MRI can be used as a primary diagnostic tool in enrolling patients for active surveillance and as an alternative to biopsy (Fig. 2.6). Therefore, the European Association of Urology guidelines recommend MRI for patients on active surveillance even after the initial biopsy [21].

Role of MRI After Radical Treatment

Elevation in PSA is the marker used to determine biochemical recurrence in patients with prostate cancer after curative intent treatment, whether surgery, external beam radiotherapy, or interstitial prostate brachytherapy, with variable thresholds for recurrence depending on the treatment received. However, while elevation in PSA constitutes biochemical recurrence, it does not provide knowledge regarding the disease site or whether there is local recurrence, distant metastasis, or both. Of note, while PI-RADS is not applicable in the posttreatment setting, a higher PI-RADS version 2 score at

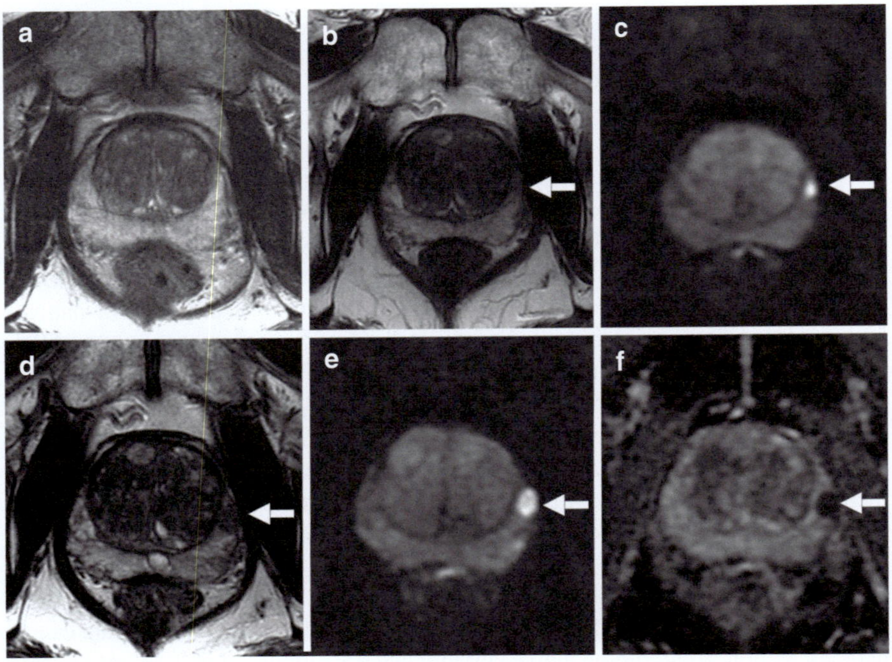

Fig. 2.6 Tumor progression after active surveillance. Prostate MRI in a 66-year-old patient with Gleason 3 + 3 prostate cancer. Baseline MRI: T2WI (**a**) shows no dominant lesion. MRI 3 years later: T2WI (**b**) shows a subtle T2 hypointense lesion in the left peripheral zone (arrow) with corresponding diffusion restriction on DWI (**c**). Subsequent biopsy revealed Gleason 3 + 3 disease and the patient stayed on active surveillance. MRI 4 years later: T2WI (**d**) revealed increase in size of the left peripheral zone lesion (arrow) with diffusion restriction on DWI (**e**) and ADC images (**f**). Subsequent prostatectomy showed Gleason 4 + 5 disease

primary staging is associated with a higher risk of biochemical recurrence, predominantly after radical prostatectomy [22]. Local recurrence after radical prostatectomy most commonly occurs at the vesicourethral anastomosis, followed by the bladder neck [23]. MRI of the treated prostate or prostatectomy bed provides high soft tissue resolution allowing for the detection of local recurrence. MRI sequences used in the posttreatment setting include T2WI, DWI, and DCE, with DCE being the most reliable sequence for detecting local recurrence [24]. Post radical prostatectomy, DCE has a pooled sensitivity of 85% and a specificity of 95%. However, after radiation therapy, the pooled sensitivity and specificity of DCE are 90% and 81%, respectively [25].

The normal appearance of the post-prostatectomy bed on T1WI and T2WI might include linear bands of low signal intensity at the site of vesicourethral anastomosis and anterior to the rectal wall due to fibrosis. There is no enhancement of the prostatic bed in the arterial phase, while subtle homogeneous enhancement can sometimes be seen in the venous phase on DCE-MRI [26]. This should be distinguished from local disease recurrence, which has characteristic intermediate signal intensity on T2WI, increased signal intensity on DWI, and avid heterogeneous enhancement in the arterial phase (Fig. 2.7) [26]. However, surgical clip susceptibility artifacts

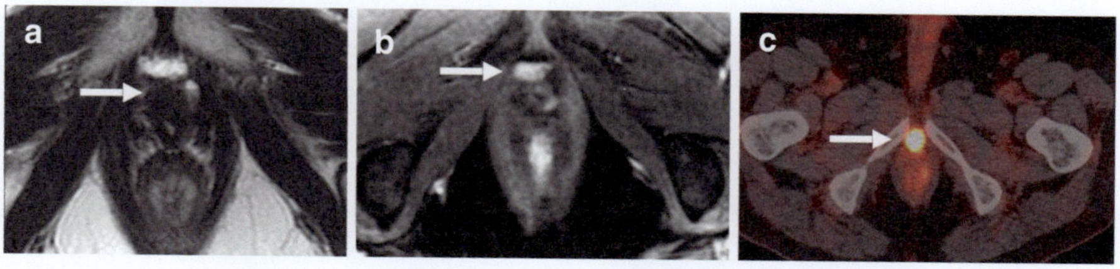

Fig. 2.7 Recurrent tumor after prostatectomy. Pelvic MRI in a 45-year-old patient, 6 years after prostatectomy for a Gleason 4 + 5 tumor. Axial T2WI (**a**) shows a low signal lesion (arrow) anterior to the vesicourethral anastomosis with corresponding early enhancement on contrast-enhanced T1WI (**b**). Gallium-68 PSMA PET/CT (**c**) reveals a corresponding tracer-avid lesion (arrow), consistent with tumor recurrence. Again, this case highlights the importance of administration of intravenous contrast in the posttreatment setting and the correlation between the existing modalities to achieve a proper diagnosis

can limit the evaluation of the surgical bed on MRI, especially on DWI [27]. In the proctectomy bed, residual prostate gland tissue may mimic disease recurrence. The residual gland appears as soft tissue with an intermediate-low signal on T1WI and T2WI, invariably at the site of anastomosis. However, the enhancement pattern on DCE-MRI can help distinguish the two entities, as recurrence typically demonstrates avid and heterogeneous enhancement during the arterial phase compared with the residual prostate gland which often uniformly enhances during the venous phase. The imaging features, alongside a lack of a complete PSA drop in these patients with residual tissue, can guide diagnosis [26]. Remnant seminal vesicles are seen in up to 20% of cases, where typically the lateral tips are identified. Remnant tissue has characteristic lobulated high signal intensity on T2WI; however, it is subject to distortion and scarring postoperatively, becoming low signal on T2WI [27].

For patients treated with radiation therapy, expected morphological changes of the treated prostate include radiation-induced inflammation, loss of normal zonal differentiation, and glandular atrophy. These changes make it challenging to distinguish disease recurrence from irradiated tissue; however, the early enhancement of recurrent tumor on DCE-MRI can help determine recurrence even at a low serum PSA level below 2.0 ng/mL (Fig. 2.8). Therefore, it is paramount to perform multiparametric MRI in this circumstance with the administration of intravenous contrast. The homogeneous early enhancement of tumor recurrence contrasts with the slow, progressive enhancement pattern of radiation-induced fibrosis [28]. Moreover, the site of signal abnormality and knowledge of the original tumor location is pertinent since there is a high propensity for recurrence at the original tumor bed after radiation therapy.

MRI can also be used to evaluate treatment responses for patients treated with androgen deprivation therapy. MRI findings for treatment response assessment include the change in prostate volume, tumor size, and decreased tumor vascularity which is linked to a decrease in serum PSA level [29]. The increasing mean ADC value is also correlated with decreasing serum PSA levels. Additionally, the correlation between ADC value and treatment response has been investigated. After treatment, the mean ADC

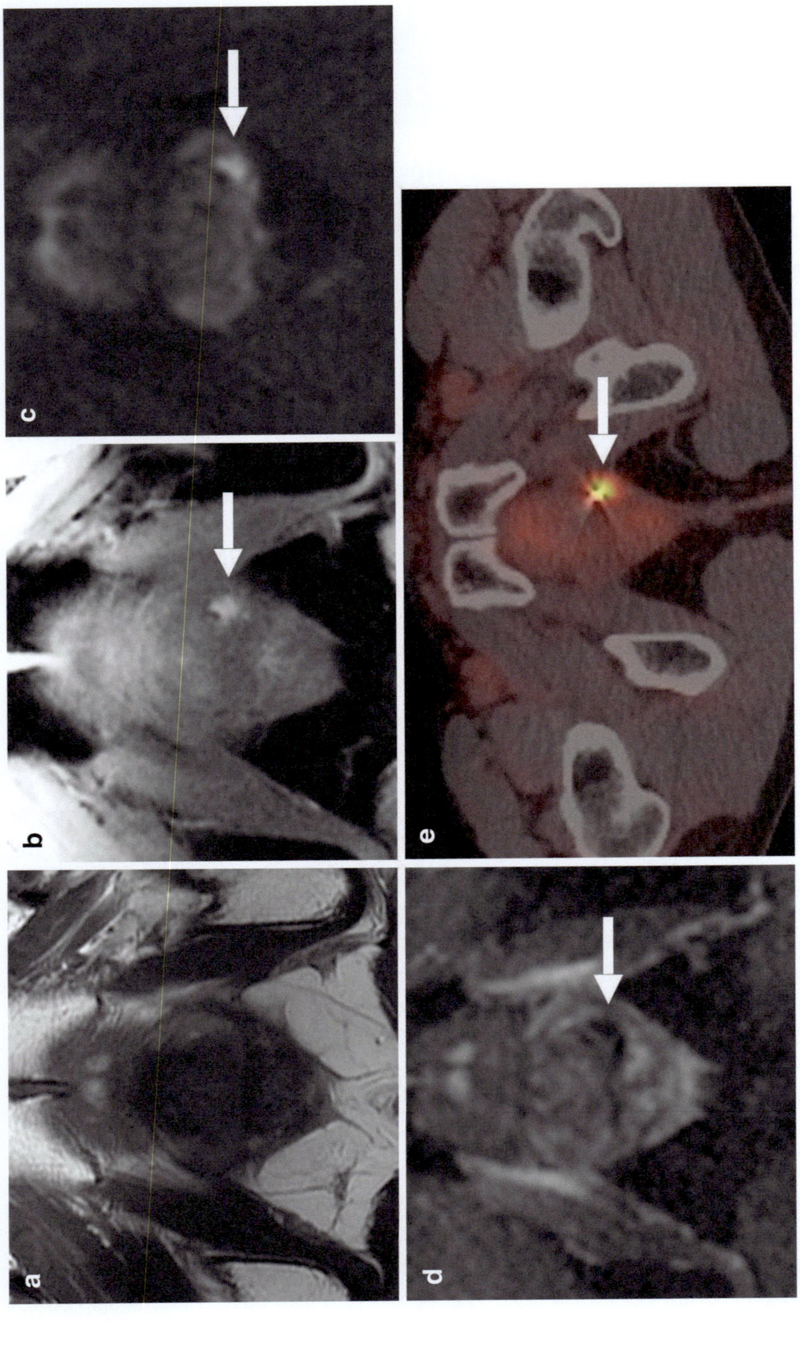

Fig. 2.8 Recurrent tumor after radiation. Prostate MRI in a 68-year-old patient, 6 years after radiation therapy for a Gleason 3 + 4 tumor. T2WI (**a**) shows a diffuse low signal throughout the prostate gland, consistent with posttreatment change. Contrast-enhanced T1WI (**b**) shows an enhancing lesion (arrow) in the left posterior mid-gland peripheral zone with corresponding restricted signal on DWI (**c**) and ADC map (**d**). Gallium-68 PSMA PET/CT (**e**) reveals a tracer-avid lesion (arrow), consistent with tumor recurrence. This case highlights the importance of administration of intravenous contrast in the posttreatment setting for proper evaluation

value of the tumor increases compared with the pretreatment value (1060×10^{-6} mm^2/s versus 780×10^{-6} mm^2/s) [30]. Further studies are needed to assess if this will help predict pathological downstaging or even pathological complete response.

Focal therapies, such as cryotherapy, high-intensity focused ultrasound, and photodynamic treatment, result in tumor necrosis [31]. Therefore, patients with low- to intermediate-risk, organ-confined prostate cancer can benefit from focal therapies and avoid morbidities associated with radical therapies. Expected MRI findings posttreatment include a focal non-enhancing area at the tumor bed. In contrast, tumor recurrence is typically seen as an early enhancing focal lesion with restricted diffusion in or adjacent to the originally treated tumor [32, 33].

Imaging in the Management of Biochemical Recurrence

Imaging plays a fundamental role in the management of biochemical recurrence as it provides an accurate and objective assessment of disease burden. This is pertinent since early diagnosis of biochemical recurrence allows site-directed therapy, particularly in oligometastatic disease [34]. Oligo-recurrent disease often has a distinctly less aggressive course and may benefit from metastasis-directed therapy, which improves progression-free survival related to biochemical recurrence [35].

The role of imaging in the management of biochemical recurrence varies depending on the type of imaging modality. TRUS and MRI are, for example, only able to evaluate local recurrence because of their limited coverage of the treated prostate and pelvic lymph nodes. Whole-body MRI allows the detection and quantification of distant disease metastases, which further aids in tailoring treatment by differentiating oligometastatic from poly-metastatic disease. The evolving whole-body MRI protocols are optimized to detect various metastases, including spread to the lymph nodes, bone, and visceral organs such as the liver and lung. Whole-body MRI has demonstrated superior performance in detecting osseous lesions compared with bone scintigraphy and radiography [36]. Meanwhile, positron emission tomography (PET) imaging, whether combined with computed tomography (CT) or MRI as hybrid PET/CT or PET/MRI, is superior for evaluating extraprostatic disease, particularly with emerging novel radiotracers such as ^{11}C-choline or prostate-specific membrane antigen (PSMA), which will be discussed.

CT and MRI

CT and MRI are commonly used to evaluate metastatic spread to the lymph nodes, the bone, and visceral organs. CT of the pelvis is used to evaluate local recurrence and metastatic spread to the lymph nodes; however, it has limited value for detecting local recurrence unless the tumor is large (>2.0 cm) [37], and it has a relatively low sensitivity of 42% for detecting nodal metastases since CT-based assessment relies on morphologic assessment and size criteria [38, 39]. These limitations result in significant staging and diagnosis delays, which ultimately negatively affects treatment planning, especially when PSA level is less than 5 ng/mL. Meanwhile, CT of the chest is used to evaluate thoracic metastases involving the lung, pleura, and mediastinum.

For osseous metastasis, CT might be useful in detecting sclerotic bone and visceral metastases; however, bone scintigraphy and MRI remain superior for establishing diagnosis and follow-up. Of note, the "flare" phenomenon refers to the appearance of worsening disease on imaging after the initiation of androgen deprivation therapy or chemotherapy, despite actual overall clinical improvement. This phenomenon is attributed to the increased osteoblastic reaction of new bone formation and appears as increased bone sclerosis on CT and MRI [40]. The incidence of this phenomenon peaks during the first 6 weeks after treatment initiation.

Two evaluation criteria are available for evaluating prostate cancer disease progression on imaging in clinical trials—the Response Evaluation Criteria in Solid Tumors (RECIST) version 1.1, which is used for soft tissue disease, and the Prostate Cancer Clinical Trials Working Group 2 criteria, which is used for osseous disease. Disease progression for osseous lesions needs to be confirmed based on two scans, with a time interval of 6 or more weeks between the scans [41].

Bone Scintigraphy

Bone scintigraphy involves the use of the radiotracer ^{99}mTc-methylene diphosphonate (^{99}mTc-MDP) to detect osseous metastases (Figs. 2.3 and 2.5). Although it is widely available and regularly used for posttreatment follow-up evaluation, it has a relatively low sensitivity and specificity of 79–82% for detecting osseous metastases compared with other imaging modalities. This is particularly evident in asymptomatic patients and when serum PSA is below 7 ng/mL [42].

Radiotracer uptake on bone scintigraphy depends on the degree of reactionary osteoblastic activity induced by tumor cells rather than the tumor cells themselves. Bone scans can potentially miss osteolytic bone marrow metastases or small osteoblastic metastases that do not induce osteoblastic reaction sufficient for detection, resulting in significant underestimation of disease burden.

Additionally, in the scenario of the "flare" phenomenon, the osteoblastic effect of the healing bone results in increased tracer uptake after treatment initiation; thus, radiological correlation with clinical symptoms and PSA levels is mandatory to distinguish between response to treatment and disease progression [40].

Finally, benign osteoblastic conditions such as fractures, Paget disease, and degenerative changes can result in increased tracer uptake, mimicking metastases [43, 44]. In these cases, knowledge of the expected patterns of radiotracer uptake and correlation with other imaging modalities and PSA levels will be helpful in distinguishing between multiple possible entities.

PET and PET/CT

PET imaging is superior for the evaluation of extraprostatic disease. The emergence of novel radiotracers, e.g., choline and PSMA, has created a paradigm shift in managing patients with prostate cancer, particularly those with recurrent biochemical prostate cancer. The use of such novel tracers allows for early detection of recurrence even at atypical sites such as the pancreas or adrenal gland, allowing site-directed metastasis.

^{18}F-FDG ^{18}F-fluorodeoxyglucose (^{18}F-FDG) is a glucose analog taken up by tumors with a high rate of metabolism. The upregulation of tumor cells' transporter proteins results in increased ^{18}F-FDG uptake. Despite its advantages and wide use in PET imaging, ^{18}F-FDG PET is limited in patients with prostate cancer due to the dependence of prostate cancer on non-glucose metabolic pathways such as fatty acids or fructose [45]. Moreover, the high renal excretion and urinary bladder accumulation of ^{18}F-FDG may hinder the detection of local recurrence [46]. ^{18}F-FDG uptake can be seen in patients with aggressive or rapidly progressive prostate cancer, and the degree of uptake is related to the degree of PSA level elevation. Therefore, the use of ^{18}F-FDG is limited to certain subsets of patients [47, 48].

^{18}F-NaF ^{18}F-sodium fluoride (^{18}F-NaF) is an analog of the hydroxyl group in hydroxyapatite bone crystals [49]. It has rapid renal clearance and minimal protein affinity, making it an ideal tracer for detecting bone metastases, especially in obese patients [49, 50]. ^{18}F-NaF PET/CT is more accurate compared with bone scintigraphy since it provides superior images shortly after administration. However, its accuracy is inadequate for detecting metastases to soft tissues or lymph nodes.

^{18}F-fluciclovine ^{18}F-fluciclovine is also known as anti-1-amino-3-^{18}F--fluorocyclobutane-1–carboxylic acid (FACBC). It is a US Food and Drug Administration-approved, radiolabeled, non-natural amino acid that targets amino acid transporters (LAT1 and ASCT2). ^{18}F-fluciclovine has relatively low early urinary excretion, which has led to its utilization in cases with urogenital and pelvic malignancies [51].

In general, ^{18}F-fluciclovine PET/CT has a reported mean detection rate of 47% for biochemical recurrence and a high positive predictive value of 92.3–95.7% for recurrent extraprostatic disease [52]. In addition, ^{18}F-fluciclovine has the advantage of being widely available in the United States. Similar to other radiotracers, common pathologies detected include inflammatory or infectious processes and other malignancies such as lymphoma, which can have avid radiotracer uptake.

PSMA PSMA is a transmembrane enzyme (folate hydrolase I or glutamate carboxypeptidase II) that both the prostate cancer itself and the neovasculature of malignant cells highly express. In addition, its expression is associated with tumor grade and disease prognosis (Figs. 2.9 and 2.10) [53].

^{68}Ga-PSMA-11 was the first FDA-approved PSMA agent in 2020 for research purposes [54]. This was followed by the approval of ^{18}F-labeled (2S)-2-[[(1S)-1-carboxy-5- [(6- (^{18} F) fluoranylpyridine-3-carbonyl) amino] pentyl]carbamoylamino] pentanedioic acid (^{18} F-DCFPyL) as the first commercially available PSMA PET agent for imaging of prostate cancer. ^{68}Ga-PSMA-11 has consistently shown to be superior to conventional imaging and other radiotracers [55–59]. Meanwhile,

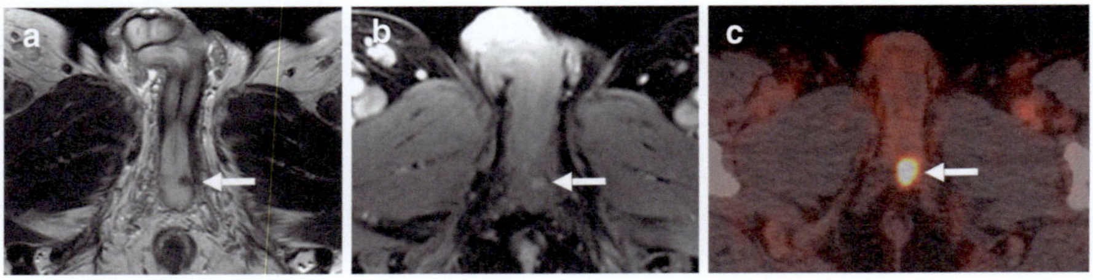

Fig. 2.9 Recurrent tumor after prostatectomy. Pelvic MRI in a 75-year-old patient with rising PSA 6 years after prostatectomy. T2WI (**a**) shows a hypointense nodule (arrow) in the penile bulb on the left side with early enhancement on contrast-enhanced T1WI (**b**) and Gallium-68 PSMA uptake (**c**), consistent with metastasis

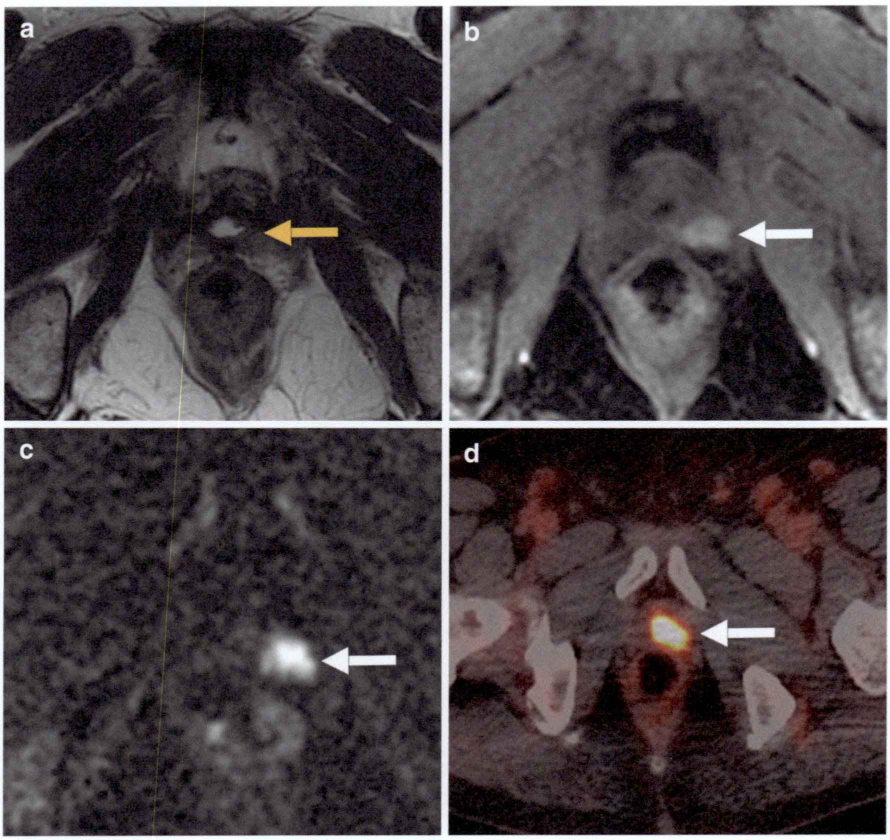

Fig. 2.10 Recurrent tumor post-focal therapy. Prostate MRI in a 68-year-old patient with Gleason 3 + 4 prostate cancer with high-intensity focused ultrasound (HIFU) 11 years prior. T2WI (**a**) shows a markedly small prostate gland with a dilated prostatic urethra (yellow arrow). Contrast-enhanced T1WI (**b**) shows an early enhancing lesion (arrow) in the left prostate gland with corresponding diffusion restriction on DWI (**c**) and tracer uptake on subsequent gallium-68 PSMA PET/CT (**d**). Subsequent biopsy showed recurrent disease

several prospective studies, including the CONDOR and OSPREY multicenter studies, have reported high predictive value and specificity of ^{18}F-DCFPyL, supporting its potential value in diagnosing suspected recurrence [60, 61].

PSMA could also be a useful diagnostic marker and theranostic agent in the setting of tumor-targeted radionuclide therapy with actinium-225 (225Ac-PSMA) and lutetium-labeled PSMA ligand ^{177}Lu-PSMA-617 [62].

Choline Choline is a substrate precursor involved in cell membrane synthesis and transmembrane signaling. Malignant cells have high cell membrane synthesis, which results in increased choline uptake. In addition, the longer half-life of ^{18}F-choline compared to ^{11}C-choline (110 vs 20 minutes) allows for its wider distribution and negates the need for an on-site cyclotron, which is required to generate ^{11}C-choline [63]. However, the high urinary excretion of ^{18}F-choline impedes the diagnostic accuracy for pelvic juxta-renal or ureteric metastasis detection.

^{11}C-choline PET has a high diagnostic accuracy compared to conventional imaging, significantly impacting patient management by allowing personalized treatments [63, 64]. Moreover, it can detect recurrence in patients on active surveillance with low PSA levels of 0.1 ng/mL [65].

Similar to other tracers, ^{11}C-choline can accumulate and show increased uptake in sites of inflammatory activity, benign tumors, and other primary malignancies [66]. Correlation with clinical history and histopathology is of prime importance in such cases.

PET/MRI

The emerging PET/MRI technology combines the strengths of PET with concurrent MRI. The superior anatomic characterization and recurrence localization of PET/MRI make it a valuable tool for primary tumor detection and staging as well as early detection of disease recurrence [67]. In addition, PET/MRI can impact clinical decision and management; studies have shown that PSMA PET/MRI can alter restaging clinical management in up to 75% of patients with prostate cancer. However, more studies are required to ascertain the value of PET/MRI [68, 69].

The functional information provided by PET novel tracers such as ^{11}C-choline and PSMA-targeted radioligands can detect disease in morphologically normal and subcentimeter nodes. Compared with PET/CT, PET/MRI has higher detection rates for local recurrence at the surgical bed, which is frequently obscured by tracer excretion on PET/CT [67, 70, 71].

Radiomics and Artificial Intelligence

Radiomics is an emerging noninvasive tool that extracts and evaluates predictive signatures on imaging that are not perceived by the human eye and are believed to have value in serving as novel biomarkers to aid in screening, disease evaluation, treatment response assessment, risk stratification, and recurrence detection [72].

In the management of prostate cancer, radiomics is a promising quantitative tool. Multiple fully- or semiautomated models have been published to date for various clinical scenarios and based on multiple imaging modalities, incorporating radiomic features only or radiomic features combined with clinical information; however, these models remain confined to the research realm [72].

The majority of radiomic studies in prostate cancer have been based on MRI, with models developed for initial prostate cancer detection, stratification of lesions into low- or high-risk categories, prediction of Gleason score, and treatment planning and assessment [73–77]. In one study, a model incorporating radiomic features from MRI combined with clinical information and PSA level was developed, which showed potential to decrease the number of patients needing a prostate biopsy by 18.4% [78]. In another study, the addition of radiomic features improved the performance of PI-RADS scores for prostate cancer in the peripheral zone (area under the curve (AUC) = 0.983) versus the transitional zone (AUC = 0.968) [79]. While only a few studies have focused on detecting extracapsular extension using radiomic features, promising results have been reported; for example, one study reported that the radiomic signature yielded a sensitivity of 75% and an AUC of 0.90 and 0.88 in the training and validation cohorts, respectively, outperforming radiologists who had a sensitivity of 46.88–50.00% ($p < 0.05$) in the same cohorts [80]. In post-radiotherapy settings, radiomic features have been extracted from the ADC map and T2WI, since changes in the tumor ADC mean value in response to treatment are also reflected in changes in first- and second-order radiomic features [81]. Similarly, radiomic features extracted from T2WI and ADC for response assessment can help differentiate tumor from normal tissue; this is paramount when planning for radiotherapy post neoadjuvant androgen deprivation therapy [82, 83]. For the prediction of biochemical recurrence, published models are available for post-radical prostatectomy and radiation therapy settings. These prediction models are based on radiomic features extracted from pretreatment MRI, some also incorporating clinical information [72, 84–86].

Besides radiomic features extracted from MRI, radiomic features have also been extracted from PSMA PET/CT for prostate cancer staging, including the evaluation of nodal and distant metastasis, with radiomic models showing comparable performance to experienced radiologists in classifying hotspots with high precision [87, 88].

TRUS-based radiomics have also been studied, especially as US is a widely available imaging modality that is relatively more affordable and less expensive than other imaging modalities. One of the highest-performing published models used multiparametric (using B-mode, shear-wave elastography, and DCE ultrasound) radiomic-based classification, which yielded an AUC of 0.90 [72, 89].

While the initial results are promising, most of these models are based on manual segmentation and selection of the region of interest. Additionally, most of these studies are retrospective in nature. Therefore, further studies are needed to test these models' robustness and reproducibility before being integrated into clinical practice.

Take-Home Message

The authors very thoroughly highlighted the landscape of imaging in diagnosis, treatment, and surveillance of prostate cancer, covering MRI, CT, PET, radiomics, and artificial intelligence. We believe that prostate MRI should be considered an extension of the physical exam of any man presenting for diagnosis and treatment of prostate cancer. MRI not only gives vital information about the size of the gland and any suspicious lesion, but it can also help dictate the degree of nerve sparing at the time of prostatectomy by showing areas of extraprostatic extension or neurovascular bundle involvement. While not typically used for identification of local lymph node metastasis, occasionally enlarged pelvic lymph nodes can at times be seen and influence decisions for further staging imaging and/or lymph node dissection template at the time of surgery.

Recently, PSMA PET has been fervently studied in the space of primary diagnosis as well as biochemically recurrent prostate cancer. Further studies are needed to see whether the combination of PSMA PET with MRI can obviate the need for prostate biopsy altogether.

References

1. Turkbey B, et al. Prostate imaging reporting and data system version 2.1: 2019 update of prostate imaging reporting and data system version 2. Eur Urol. 2019;76(3):340–51.
2. Bhavsar A, Verma S. Anatomic imaging of the prostate. Biomed Res Int. 2014;2014:728539.
3. Ryan S, et al. Anatomy for diagnostic imaging. 3rd ed. Edinburgh/New York: Saunders/Elsevier; 2011, vi, 337 pages: illustrations
4. Janus C, Lippert M. Benign prostatic hyperplasia: appearance on magnetic resonance imaging. Urology. 1992;40(6):539–41.
5. Villeirs GM, et al. Magnetic resonance imaging anatomy of the prostate and periprostatic area: a guide for radiotherapists. Radiother Oncol. 2005;76(1):99–106.
6. Harada T, et al. Five-point Likert scaling on MRI predicts clinically significant prostate carcinoma. BMC Urol. 2015;15:91.
7. Sakala MD, Dyer RB, Tappouni R. The "erased charcoal" sign. Abdom Radiol. 2017;42(3):981–2.
8. Yu J, et al. Diagnosis of typical and atypical transition zone prostate cancer and its mimics at multiparametric prostate MRI. Br J Radiol. 2017;90(1073):20160693.
9. Zhang F, et al. Accuracy of multiparametric magnetic resonance imaging for detecting extracapsular extension in prostate cancer: a systematic review and meta-analysis. Br J Radiol. 2019;92(1104):20190480.
10. Mehralivand S, et al. A grading system for the assessment of risk of extraprostatic extension of prostate cancer at multiparametric MRI. Radiology. 2019;290(3):709–19.
11. Ghafoor S, Burger IA, Vargas AH. Multimodality imaging of prostate cancer. J Nucl Med. 2019;60(10):1350–8.
12. Van Nieuwenhove S, et al. Whole-body magnetic resonance imaging for prostate cancer assessment: current status and future directions. J Magn Reson Imaging. 2022;55(3):653–80.
13. Turkbey B, Choyke PL. Birth of a standard: MET-RADS-P for metastatic prostate cancer. Nat Rev Urol. 2016;13(10):568–70.
14. Padhani AR, et al. METastasis reporting and data system for prostate cancer: practical guidelines for acquisition, interpretation, and reporting of whole-body magnetic resonance imaging-based evaluations of multiorgan involvement in advanced prostate cancer. Eur Urol. 2017;71(1):81–92.

15. Woo S, et al. Comparison of magnetic resonance imaging-stratified clinical pathways and systematic transrectal ultrasound-guided biopsy pathway for the detection of clinically significant prostate cancer: a systematic review and meta-analysis of randomized controlled trials. Eur Urol Oncol. 2019;2(6):605–16.
16. Bhat KRS, et al. Magnetic resonance imaging-guided prostate biopsy-a review of literature. Asian J Urol. 2021;8(1):105–16.
17. Moldovan PC, et al. What is the negative predictive value of multiparametric magnetic resonance imaging in excluding prostate cancer at biopsy? A systematic review and meta-analysis from the European Association of Urology Prostate Cancer Guidelines Panel. Eur Urol. 2017;72(2):250–66.
18. Ahmed HU, et al. Diagnostic accuracy of multi-parametric MRI and TRUS biopsy in prostate cancer (PROMIS): a paired validating confirmatory study. Lancet. 2017;389(10071):815–22.
19. Carroll PR, et al. NCCN guidelines insights: prostate cancer early detection, version 2.2016. J Natl Compr Canc Netw. 2016;14(5):509–19.
20. Sklinda K, Mruk B, Walecki J. Active surveillance of prostate cancer using multiparametric magnetic resonance imaging: a review of the current role and future perspectives. Med Sci Monit. 2020;26:e920252.
21. EAU Guidelines. Edn. presented at the EAU Annual Congress. Amsterdam; 2022. Available from: https://uroweb.org/guidelines/prostate-cancer/chapter/citation-information.
22. Rajwa P, et al. The prognostic association of prostate MRI PI-RADS v2 assessment category and risk of biochemical recurrence after definitive local therapy for prostate cancer: a systematic review and meta-analysis. J Urol. 2021;206(3):507–16.
23. Bhargava P, et al. Imaging biochemical recurrence after prostatectomy: where are we headed? AJR Am J Roentgenol. 2020;214(6):1248–58.
24. Panebianco V, et al. Prostate cancer recurrence after radical prostatectomy: the role of 3-T diffusion imaging in multi-parametric magnetic resonance imaging. Eur Radiol. 2013;23(6):1745–52.
25. Wu LM, et al. Role of magnetic resonance imaging in the detection of local prostate cancer recurrence after external beam radiotherapy and radical prostatectomy. Clin Oncol (R Coll Radiol). 2013;25(4):252–64.
26. Allen SD, Thompson A, Sohaib SA. The normal post-surgical anatomy of the male pelvis following radical prostatectomy as assessed by magnetic resonance imaging. Eur Radiol. 2008;18(6):1281–91.
27. Sella T, Schwartz LH, Hricak H. Retained seminal vesicles after radical prostatectomy: frequency, MRI characteristics, and clinical relevance. AJR Am J Roentgenol. 2006;186(2):539–46.
28. Kim CK, et al. Prostate MR imaging at 3T using a phased-arrayed coil in predicting locally recurrent prostate cancer after radiation therapy: preliminary experience. Abdom Imaging. 2010;35(2):246–52.
29. Padhani AR, et al. Effects of androgen deprivation on prostatic morphology and vascular permeability evaluated with MR imaging. Radiology. 2001;218(2):365–74.
30. Kim AY, et al. Diffusion-weighted imaging to evaluate for changes from androgen deprivation therapy in prostate cancer. AJR Am J Roentgenol. 2014;203(6):W645–50.
31. van der Poel HG, et al. Focal therapy in primary localised prostate cancer: the European Association of Urology Position in 2018. Eur Urol. 2018;74(1):84–91.
32. Ghafoor S, et al. Magnetic resonance imaging of the prostate after focal therapy with high-intensity focused ultrasound. Abdom Radiol (NY). 2020;45(11):3882–95.
33. Lotte R, et al. Multiparametric MRI for suspected recurrent prostate cancer after HIFU: is DCE still needed? Eur Radiol. 2018;28(9):3760–9.
34. Ost P, et al. Surveillance or metastasis-directed therapy for oligometastatic prostate cancer recurrence: a prospective, randomized, multicenter phase II trial. J Clin Oncol. 2018;36(5):446–53.
35. Ost P, et al. Surveillance or metastasis-directed therapy for oligometastatic prostate cancer recurrence (STOMP): five-year results of a randomized phase II trial. J Clin Oncol. 2020;38(6_suppl):10.

36. Lecouvet FE, et al. Magnetic resonance imaging of the axial skeleton for detecting bone metastases in patients with high-risk prostate cancer: diagnostic and cost-effectiveness and comparison with current detection strategies. J Clin Oncol. 2007;25(22):3281–7.
37. Barwick TD, Castellucci P. Invited commentary: changing landscape of imaging in recurrent prostate cancer. Radiographics. 2020;40(3):727–30.
38. Abuzallouf S, Dayes I, Lukka H. Baseline staging of newly diagnosed prostate cancer: a summary of the literature. J Urol. 2004;171(6 Pt 1):2122–7.
39. Hovels AM, et al. The diagnostic accuracy of CT and MRI in the staging of pelvic lymph nodes in patients with prostate cancer: a meta-analysis. Clin Radiol. 2008;63(4):387–95.
40. Conteduca V, et al. Flare phenomenon in prostate cancer: recent evidence on new drugs and next generation imaging. Ther Adv Med Oncol. 2021;13:1758835920987654.
41. Bryce AH, et al. Radiographic progression with nonrising PSA in metastatic castration-resistant prostate cancer: post hoc analysis of PREVAIL. Prostate Cancer Prostatic Dis. 2017;20(2):221–7.
42. Shen G, et al. Comparison of choline-PET/CT, MRI, SPECT, and bone scintigraphy in the diagnosis of bone metastases in patients with prostate cancer: a meta-analysis. Skeletal Radiol. 2014;43(11):1503–13.
43. Agrawal A, et al. Metastatic mimics on bone scan: “All that glitters is not metastatic”. Indian J Nucl Med. 2016;31(3):185–90.
44. Fukushi K, et al. Paget’s disease mimicking metastatic prostate cancer on bone scan image: a case report. Hinyokika Kiyo. 2013;59(4):247–50.
45. Liu Y, Zuckier LS, Ghesani NV. Dominant uptake of fatty acid over glucose by prostate cells: a potential new diagnostic and therapeutic approach. Anticancer Res. 2010;30(2):369–74.
46. Patel DN, Karsh LI, Daskivich TJ. Next-generation imaging in localized high-risk prostate cancer. Prostate Cancer Prostatic Dis. 2021;24(3):585–6.
47. Schoder H, et al. 2-[F-18]Fluoro-2-deoxyglucose positron emission tomography for the detection of disease in patients with prostate-specific antigen relapse after radical prostatectomy. Clin Cancer Res. 2005;11(13):4761–9.
48. Jadvar H. Is there use for FDG-PET in prostate cancer? Semin Nucl Med. 2016;46(6):502–6.
49. Czernin J, Satyamurthy N, Schiepers C. Molecular mechanisms of bone 18F-NaF deposition. J Nucl Med. 2010;51(12):1826–9.
50. Usmani S, et al. F-18-NaF PET/CT of obese patients on a lutetium-yttrium oxyorthosilicate PET/CT system: patient dosimetry, optimization of injected activity, and acquisition time. J Nucl Med Technol. 2021;49(2):150–5.
51. Kim EH, et al. Prostate cancer recurrence in patients with negative or equivocal conventional imaging: a role for F-18-fluciclovine-PET/CT in delineating sites of recurrence and identifying patients with oligometastatic disease. Urol Oncol. 2021;39(6):365.e9.
52. Calais J, Ceci F, Eiber M. F-18-fluciclovine PET-CT and Ga-68-PSMA-11 PET-CT in patients with early biochemical recurrence after prostatectomy: a prospective, single-centre, single-arm, comparative imaging trial (vol 20, pg 1286, 2019). Lancet Oncol. 2020;21(6):E304.
53. Lawhn-Heath C, et al. Prostate-specific membrane antigen PET in prostate cancer. Radiology. 2021;299(2):248–60.
54. Geoffrey Johnson, M.C. Expanded access [Ga-68] PSMA-11 PET imaging. 2021. Available from: https://clinicaltrials.gov/ct2/show/NCT04800068.
55. Dietlein M, et al. Comparison of [F-18]DCFPyL and [Ga-68]Ga-PSMA-HBED-CC for PSMA-PET imaging in patients with relapsed prostate cancer. Mol Imaging Biol. 2015;17(4):575–84.
56. Fowler M. FDA approves 18F-DCFPyL as first PSMA PET imaging agent available for prostate cancer. 2021. Available from: https://www.cancernetwork.com/view/fda-approves-18f-dcfpyl-as-first-psma-pet-imaging-agent-available-for-prostate-cancer.
57. Hope TA, et al. Metaanalysis of Ga-68-PSMA-11 PET accuracy for the detection of prostate cancer validated by histopathology. J Nucl Med. 2019;60(6):786–93.
58. Kranzbuhler B, et al. Detection rate and localization of prostate cancer recurrence using Ga-68-PSMA-11 PET/MRI in patients with low PSA values <= 0.5 ng/mL. J Nucl Med. 2020;61(2):194–201.

59. Alonso O, et al. Ga-68-PSMA and C-11-choline comparison using a tri-modality PET/CT-MRI (3.0 T) system with a dedicated shuttle. Eur J Hybrid Imaging. 2018;2(1):9.
60. Pienta KJ, et al. A phase 2/3 prospective multicenter study of the diagnostic accuracy of prostate specific membrane antigen PET/CT with (18)F-DCFPyL in prostate cancer patients (OSPREY). J Urol. 2021;206(1):52–61.
61. Morris MJ, et al. Diagnostic performance of F-18-DCFPyL-PET/CT in men with biochemically recurrent prostate cancer: results from the CONDOR phase III, multicenter study. Clin Cancer Res. 2021;27(13):3674–82.
62. Kratochwil C, et al. [(1)(7)(7)Lu]Lutetium-labelled PSMA ligand-induced remission in a patient with metastatic prostate cancer. Eur J Nucl Med Mol Imaging. 2015;42(6):987–8.
63. Mitchell CR, et al. Operational characteristics of (11)c-choline positron emission tomography/computerized tomography for prostate cancer with biochemical recurrence after initial treatment. J Urol. 2013;189(4):1308–13.
64. Ceci F, et al. Impact of 11C-choline PET/CT on clinical decision making in recurrent prostate cancer: results from a retrospective two-Centre trial (vol 41, pg 2222, 2014). Eur J Nucl Med Mol Imaging. 2014;41(12):2359.
65. Garg I, et al. (11)C-choline positron emission tomography/computed tomography for detection of disease relapse in patients with history of biochemically recurrent prostate cancer and prostate-specific antigen </=0.1 ng/ml. J Cancer Res Ther. 2021;17(2):358–65.
66. Welle CL, et al. (1)(1)C-choline PET/CT in recurrent prostate cancer and nonprostatic neoplastic processes. Radiographics. 2016;36(1):279–92.
67. Evangelista L, et al. PET/MRI in prostate cancer: a systematic review and meta-analysis. Eur J Nucl Med Mol Imaging. 2021;48(3):859–73.
68. Hope TA, et al. Impact of (68)Ga-PSMA-11 PET on management in patients with biochemically recurrent prostate cancer. J Nucl Med. 2017;58(12):1956–61.
69. Schiller K, et al. Patterns of failure after radical prostatectomy in prostate cancer – implications for radiation therapy planning after Ga-68-PSMA-PET imaging. Eur J Nucl Med Mol Imaging. 2017;44(10):1656–62.
70. Galgano SJ, et al. Utility of (18)F-fluciclovine PET/MRI for staging newly diagnosed high-risk prostate cancer and evaluating response to initial androgen deprivation therapy: a prospective single-arm pilot study. AJR Am J Roentgenol. 2021;217(3):720–9.
71. Souvatzoglou M, et al. Comparison of integrated whole-body [11C]choline PET/MR with PET/CT in patients with prostate cancer. Eur J Nucl Med Mol Imaging. 2013;40(10):1486–99.
72. Ferro M, et al. Radiomics in prostate cancer: an up-to-date review. Ther Adv Urol. 2022;14
73. Macomber MW, et al. Autosegmentation of prostate anatomy for radiation treatment planning using deep decision forests of radiomic features. Phys Med Biol. 2018;63(23):235002.
74. Khalvati F, et al. MPCaD: a multi-scale radiomics-driven framework for automated prostate cancer localization and detection. BMC Med Imaging. 2018;18(1):16.
75. Cuocolo R, et al. Clinically significant prostate cancer detection on MRI: a radiomic shape features study. Eur J Radiol. 2019;116:144–9.
76. Chaddad A, et al. Predicting Gleason score of prostate cancer patients using radiomic analysis. Front Oncol. 2018;8:630.
77. Chaddad A, Kucharczyk MJ, Niazi T. Multimodal radiomic features for the predicting Gleason score of prostate cancer. Cancers (Basel). 2018;10(8)
78. Qi Y, et al. Multiparametric MRI-based radiomics for prostate cancer screening with PSA in 4-10 ng/mL to reduce unnecessary biopsies. J Magn Reson Imaging. 2020;51(6):1890–9.
79. Wang J, et al. Machine learning-based analysis of MR radiomics can help to improve the diagnostic performance of PI-RADS v2 in clinically relevant prostate cancer. Eur Radiol. 2017;27(10):4082–90.
80. Ma S, et al. MRI-based radiomics signature for the preoperative prediction of extracapsular extension of prostate cancer. J Magn Reson Imaging. 2019;50(6):1914–25.
81. Lee SL, et al. Changes in apparent diffusion coefficient radiomics features during dose-painted radiotherapy and high dose rate brachytherapy for prostate cancer. Phys Imaging Radiat Oncol. 2019;9:1–6.

82. Reischauer C, et al. Texture analysis of apparent diffusion coefficient maps for treatment response assessment in prostate cancer bone metastases-a pilot study. Eur J Radiol. 2018;101:184–90.
83. Reischauer C, et al. Bone metastases from prostate cancer: assessing treatment response by using diffusion-weighted imaging and functional diffusion maps--initial observations. Radiology. 2010;257(2):523–31.
84. Zhong QZ, et al. Radiomics of multiparametric MRI to predict biochemical recurrence of localized prostate cancer after radiation therapy. Front Oncol. 2020;10:731.
85. Shiradkar R, et al. Radiomic features from pretreatment biparametric MRI predict prostate cancer biochemical recurrence: preliminary findings. J Magn Reson Imaging. 2018;48(6):1626–36.
86. Li L, et al. A novel imaging based nomogram for predicting post-surgical biochemical recurrence and adverse pathology of prostate cancer from pre-operative bi-parametric MRI. EBioMedicine. 2021;63:103163.
87. Moazemi S, et al. Machine learning facilitates hotspot classification in PSMA-PET/CT with nuclear medicine specialist accuracy. Diagnostics (Basel). 2020;10(9)
88. Erle A, et al. Evaluating a machine learning tool for the classification of pathological uptake in whole-body PSMA-PET-CT scans. Tomography. 2021;7(3):301–12.
89. Wildeboer RR, et al. Automated multiparametric localization of prostate cancer based on B-mode, shear-wave elastography, and contrast-enhanced ultrasound radiomics. Eur Radiol. 2020;30(2):806–15.

"Preoperative Assessment and Intervention: Optimizing Outcomes for Early Return of Urinary Continence and Erectile Function"

3

Christopher R. Koller, Garrett Brinkley, and Raju Thomas

Introduction

In 2022, there were around 270,000 new cases of prostate cancer and around 35,000 deaths from prostate cancer in the USA yearly [1]. Although prostate cancer is the second leading cause of cancer-related death, most men do not die from the disease [1]. In fact, more than 3.1 million men in the USA diagnosed with prostate cancer are still alive today. The National Comprehensive Cancer Network (NCCN) gives guidelines for best practices for urologists based on current literature. The risk stratification for clinically localized disease ranges from very low to very high. Options at each stage typically include active surveillance (AS), external beam radiation therapy (EBRT) or brachytherapy, and radical prostatectomy (RP) [2]. This chapter will focus on the last of these three options, RP. RP has a higher 10-year survival rate than radiation therapy for all grades of prostate cancer [3]. Factually, the number of radical prostatectomies performed in the USA has significantly decreased since 2012 [4]. This can partly be attributed to the common side effects associated with the procedure. Two of the most common side effects are stress urinary incontinence (SUI) and erectile dysfunction (ED). Although minimally invasive approaches, namely, laparoscopic and robot-assisted laparoscopic RP, have become more popular over the last decade, they face the same complication rate associated with SUI and ED. Prior to the introduction of the nerve-sparing technique described by Walsh et al. in 1982, ED was not preventable in patients undergoing RP [5]. Although the nerve-sparing technique and other recent surgical modifications have reduced some

C. R. Koller
National Cancer Institute, Bethesda, MD, USA
e-mail: christopher.koller@nih.gov

G. Brinkley · R. Thomas (✉)
Department of Urology, Tulane University School of Medicine, New Orleans, LA, USA
e-mail: gbrinkley@tulane.edu; rthomas@tulane.edu

S. Razdan, S. Razdan (eds.), *Urinary Continence and Sexual Function After Robotic Prostatectomy, Radiation, and Novel Therapies*,
https://doi.org/10.1007/978-3-031-64245-6_3

side effect profiles, it causes some patients to pause and some to deter from undergoing the procedure.

Incontinence

The most common complication from radical prostatectomy is urinary incontinence or the involuntary loss of urine. There are several different causes of incontinence affecting patients after their procedure. These include overactive, underactive, outlet obstruction, and most commonly stress urinary incontinence (SUI). Overactive bladder or urge urinary incontinence (UUI) develops in approximately one-third of patients postoperatively. Most patients have concomitant SUI with only 6–% presenting as only UUI [6–8]. Instead of overactivity, studies have also shown that around one-third of patients have detrusor underactivity that requires abdominal straining to urinate after the procedure. It is speculated that this is due to the denervation of the trigone [9]. In addition to irritating and denervating, surgery can also cause outlet obstruction. Obstruction caused by bladder neck contracture can lead to either overflow incontinence or UUI. Interestingly, patients have a higher risk of bladder neck contracture with open prostatectomy compared to robotic (2.6–9% compared to 0–2.1%) [10–12]. Whereas overactive and underactive bladder typically presents immediately post-surgery, bladder neck contractures typically present between 4 months and 1 year after surgery [13].

SUI

SUI is a common adverse effect after RP that can cause a significantly reduced quality of life. ICD-10 code N39.3 defines stress urinary incontinence as a form of urinary incontinence due to insufficient strength of the closure of the bladder. Most commonly, this is noticed with a loss of urine when the patient coughs or sneezes. Literature shows that 60–100% of patients will experience some form of SUI post operation [14]. Additionally, 75% of men with SUI 6 weeks post operation will continue to have it 12 months later [15]. Although 68% of patients become completely continent within 3 months, SUI can persist for 25% of patients post-RP [16]. The reduction in quality of life is significant enough for 6–9% of patients who undergo RP to undergo additional surgical procedures to treat postprostatectomy incontinence [16]. SUI is caused by sphincter malfunction, bladder dysfunction, or both.

Sphincter Dysfunction

Sphincter incompetence due to disruption of the sphincteric innervation, hypoperfusion, or direct damage to the sphincteric muscle is by far the most common reasons for post-prostatectomy incontinence [17–19]. This can be caused by dissection of either the muscle fibers or the nerve supply resulting in SUI [20]. From a study in 2011 by Gerullis et al. in prostatectomy cases that led to SUI, a transection of the sphincter was seen in 65% and sphincter penetration in 46%, or a combination was seen in 37%. The study also identified that in 87% of cases, the sphincter defect was localized to the lower circumference. Comparatively, in 45% of cases, a vesicourethral anastomosis stricture was identified [21]. A separate study using self-reported severe persistent incontinence due to intrinsic sphincter deficiency found that only 67% had pre-surgical urodynamic bladder dysfunction [22]. Identification of the cause of sphincter deficiency has been challenging as it may be difficult to identify intra op. Electromyography has been used to quantitatively measure the interference pattern of transected nerves/muscles [19]. Using this technique, Aanestad et al. and Liu et al. localized sphincter dysfunction to direct damage to the sphincter rather than the neurovascular bundle [23, 24].

Cadaveric dissection, ultrasound, and magnetic resonance imaging (MRI) have been used to describe normal urethral sphincter anatomy [25–27]. The urethral distance that extends from the apex of the prostate to the bulb of the penis, which is surrounded by the striated sphincter, is called the membranous urethral length [25, 27]. Although, Myers et al. termed it the sphincter urethra [26]. This segment of urethra is innervated by autonomic (somatic) branches of the pelvic plexus which runs both through the neurovascular bundle and from branches of the pudendal nerve by parasympathetic and sympathetic fibers. MRI can be used to measure the membranous urethral length (MUL, distance from the prostatic apex to the level of the urethra at the penile bulb). Preoperative MUL, post-RP MUL, and the MUL loss ratio all correlated with recovery time and level of urinary continence after RP [28–31]. A preoperative MUL that is larger than 12–14 mm is related to a more rapid return of urinary continence post-RP. However, this value has been questioned.

Studies that have evaluated anatomic pressure changes pre- and post-RP to identify the cause of SUI have not been particularly helpful. The maximal urethral closure pressure (MUCP) as defined by the maximum difference between the urethral pressure and the intravesical pressure is significantly reduced post-RP. The baseline MUCP in these studies was 73 cmH_2O (49–95cmH_2O) and decreased to 56 cmH_2O (30–83 cmH_2O) [20, 32–37]. However, this is likely more of a pre-surgical predictor as men that regained continence postoperatively have a significantly higher MUCP preoperatively. Therefore, not surprisingly, men who were able to eventually regain continence had a significantly higher MUCP at the follow-up appointments compared to those that did not [20]. An additional parameter studied is the function profile length (FPL), which is defined as the length of the urethra where the urethral pressure exceeds the intravesical pressure in women. Most studies do show that the FPL decreases post-operation, but only around one-half of studies show a significant difference between those that do and do not regain continence [33–35, 38–40].

Prior to Surgery

As with any medical intervention, evaluation for likelihood of development of incontinence post-RP starts with a history. It is recommended to obtain a patient's age, comorbidities, and medical and surgical history including diabetes, hypertension, coronary artery disease, obesity, and neurological status. As far back as 1996, linear regression models have demonstrated that significant risk factors for patients who develop urinary incontinence after radical prostatectomy include age, weight, degree of obstructive voiding symptoms, urethral length, radiation therapy, prior transurethral resection of the prostate, clinical stage and grade, intraoperative blood loss, resection of neurovascular bundles, postoperative anastomotic stricture, and technique of vesicourethral anastomosis [41]. Additionally, patients should undergo a post-void residual bladder scan, voiding diaries, and pad tests. Urodynamics and cystoscopy are only recommended prior to surgical intervention for urinary dysfunction or any incontinence pre-prostatectomy [42–44].

Pelvic floor muscle exercises (PFME) or pelvic floor muscle training (PFMT) has been shown to improve continence recovery if started 3–4 weeks prior to surgery [45–49]. Preoperative pelvic floor muscle training is easier learned in the preoperative setting as it can be difficult postoperatively due to muscle inhibition, sensory changes, urinary incontinence, and surgical pain [50]. It is the writer's opinion that pelvic floor muscle training is critically important and should be taught correctly. There are several methods proposed to teach men how to effectively contract the pelvic floor muscles. These utilize tactile, verbal, and visual cues. Additionally, biofeedback using surface electromyography can dramatically improve training. Anecdotally, a simple effective technique is to perform a digital rectal exam and tell the patient to demonstrate strong sphincter tone. This can easily teach patients the proper muscles to use in a short time. Continuing to encourage PFMT prior to and after RP is important in men regaining continence post-surgery.

Erectile Dysfunction

Despite excellent local oncologic control of prostate cancer after radical prostatectomy, the management of erectile dysfunction is often as important to patients as their cancer course. Clinicians can and should focus on the multitude of options available for optimizing the early return of sexual function, when possible, for patients.

Sexual dysfunction after radical prostatectomy is a well-established side effect, ranging from 14% to 90% in a recent meta-analysis, with younger men having a return of potency more often and earlier [51]. Aside from age, preoperative erectile function, as well as surgical technique, also plays a role in long-term sexual function outcomes. Nerve-sparing status is dependent on the preoperative presentation of each patient's prostate biopsy grade and location.

Erectile dysfunction following RP is mainly attributed to temporary cavernous nerve damage resulting in penile hypoxia, smooth muscle apoptosis, fibrosis, and veno-occlusive dysfunction [52]. Therefore, a thorough understanding of pelvic anatomy and physiology is critical to understanding and preventing ED postoperatively. In 1982, Walsh et al. located the innervation for the corpora cavernosa by studying the male fetus and newborns [5, 52]. This study and others described the cavernous nerves, which branch out from the pelvic plexus, travel outside the prostatic fascia posterolaterally, and are covered by levator fascia. The pelvic plexus is near the tip of the seminal vesicles and the anterior rectal wall. These nerves are accompanied by capsular arteries and veins that together are termed the neurovascular bundle (NVB). At the apex of the prostate, the NVB is located next to the membranous urethra at the 5 and 7 o'clock position. It is important to note that recent studies have suggested that branches of the pelvic plexus travel more anteriorly than originally thought, suggesting that the course of the cavernous nerves might differ substantially from that of the NVB. Additionally, the striated urethral muscle at the apex of the prostate can impinge on the nerve course. The complexity and locations of these nerves lend to the difficulty in avoiding damage during surgery [52, 53], especially with biopsy-proven apical prostate cancer.

Intraoperative and Postoperative Decision-Making for Managing

Early Return of Continence

In addition to erectile dysfunction, urinary incontinence is an inherent side effect for many men who undergo radical prostatectomy. Stanford et al. in "Urinary and Sexual Function After Radical Prostatectomy for Clinically Localized Prostate Cancer The Prostate Cancer Outcomes Study" found: "13.8% of men aged 75-79 years vs. 0.7%-3.6% of younger men experienced the highest level of incontinence at ≥18 months" [54]

Surgeons have considerable data available to them that may provide guidance in how to best avoid and then manage SUI in patients. Small, albeit important steps or techniques may lead to an earlier return of continence. Patel et al. describe the use of a periurethral suspension stitch during robotic prostatectomy as a method for increasing overall and speed of urinary continence. Placement of a periurethral retropubic stitch after dorsal venous complex ligation occurs between this venous complex and the urethra has overall positive results. The median interval to recovery of continence as statistically shorter compared to the non-suspension group in this randomized trial with the changes occurring most significantly after 3 months [55].

Other randomized trials looking at dissection and reconstruction techniques have been done with compelling results when looking specifically at urinary outcomes. Retzius-sparing (RS) prostatectomy is an approach that is entirely posterior and intrafascial, leaving the prevesical space untouched and undisturbed, which has led many to believe it provides a faster return of continence than does traditional robotic prostatectomy. A recent randomized controlled trial looking at the impact of the RS approach to continence after prostatectomy was published in 2017 by Dalela et al.

The authors compared urinary function bother and urinary continence in a group of 120 patients randomized to RS prostatectomy or traditional anterior prostatectomy. They found significant improvement in urinary continence rates as well as overall decreased urinary bother scores in patients who underwent RS prostatectomy [56].

Erectile Dysfunction

Penile rehabilitation is a key component of recovery for patients postoperatively in addition to the previously discussed surgical factors. First suggested by Briganti et al. in 2006, penile rehabilitation is based on the research findings that loss of daily nocturnal erections after RP leads to poor corporal oxygenation [57]. In a recent meta-analysis of randomized trials regarding penile rehabilitation strategies after prostatectomy, Motlagh et al. found pelvic floor muscle training and scheduled 100 mg of sildenafil to be associated with higher likelihood of erectile recovery [58]. Regular use of erectogenic medications after RP with the goal of speeding recovery has been demonstrated as well with one early study demonstrating higher rates of spontaneous functional erections in patients who were on penile rehabilitation protocols with oral or injectable medications [59].

Basic science literature in both animal and human models have illustrated improved oxygen delivery to tissues for patients who are on phosphodiesterase 5 inhibitors as well as a decrease in fibrosis and scarring of the penile smooth muscle, which may explain why patients on rehabilitation protocols may experience earlier return of erectile function in comparison to their counterparts who are not on medications early on [60]. Recent studies on low-intensity extracorporeal shockwave therapy for penile rehabilitation after RP have shown little benefit over sham controls [61].

Nerve-sparing prostatectomy has become the gold standard for preserving erectile function, when oncologically appropriate, after being first described in 1982 by Dr. Patrick Walsh [5]. Introduction of this surgical technique has dramatically decreased postoperative erectile dysfunction. Looking at the 2000 paper "The Prostate Cancer Outcomes Study," research found the following: "among men who were potent before surgery, the proportion of men reporting impotence at 18 or more months after surgery varied according to whether the procedure was nerve sparing (65.6% of non-nerve-sparing, 58.6% of unilateral, and 56.0% of bilateral nerve-sparing)" [54]. Other European studies suggest higher rates ranging from 54% to 90% with athermal and robotic techniques; however, the surgical approach (open vs. robotic) is a widely contested topic [62].

Erectile recovery is ultimately a multifactorial consequence of radical prostatectomy. Clinicians should be well versed in current data regarding surgical strategies for limiting sexual dysfunction, postoperative rehabilitation protocols, and counseling and using up-to-date data to counsel patients on the likelihood and timeline of convalescence.

Impact on Quality of Life

Although SUI and ED do not decrease life expectancy, they can reduce the quality of life for a patient. A decrease in quality of life can be a very subjective assessment of the difference between where someone views their life is at and where they believe it should be. Quantitative data for changes in quality of life is based on survey assessment. Several assessments exist for the quantification of current urinary symptoms and erectile dysfunction. Validated surveys are important for urologists to use to ensure improvement in symptoms pre- and postsurgical and nonsurgical therapies. Two of the more commonly utilized surveys are for lower urinary tract symptoms (LUTS) or ED. The American Urological Association Symptoms Score (AUASS), or also known as the International Prostate Symptom Score (IPSS), was originally introduced in 1992 as a symptom index specifically designed for what was called benign prostatic hyperplasia at the time [63]. The AUASS/IPSS can be used to quantify LUTS in men and can be helpful in identifying potential incontinence in men. However, it is not diagnostic for BPH or other etiologies of LUTS. Similarly, the International Index of Erectile Function (IIEF) or the Sexual Health Inventory for Men (SHIM) can quantify symptoms of erectile dysfunction [64, 65]. Although these two questionnaires are different, they have been shown to correlate for men facing erectile dysfunction post-RP [66].

Although these surveys can help quantify subjective symptoms, they do not quantify changes in quality of life. The EORTC QLC-C30 has been used to quantify the quality of life of patients post-RP [67]. The EORTC QLQ-C30 is a validated questionnaire for the quality of life of patients suffering from a malignancy. The survey contains 30 items and focuses on the physical, emotional, cognitive, and social functions of patients. Although studies in this area are very limited, literature shows that after a RP, those that experience ED can have an immediate decrease in quality of life, whereas those that have incontinence will perceive a reduced quality of life after 5 years [67, 68]. As the impact in QoL of SUI and ED may differ from patient to patient, both are important considerations for patients after RP considering the incredibly high number of patients who survive for decades after the procedure.

Conclusion

RP is an effective cure for radical prostatectomy but is plagued by side effect profiles that can reduce the quality of life for some patients. SUI and ED are common complications following RP that cannot be completely avoided. Preoperative evaluation of urinary and erectile function and preoperative counseling and expectations are critical, along with postoperative management strategies. Advances in understanding anatomy and physiology have reduced the number of patients who have had to suffer from these side effects. The literature on SUI and ED post-RP is both scant and dated. Without newer advances in the field, RP will continue to be challenged as a cure for prostate cancer.

Take-Home Message

Alexander Graham Bell once said "before anything else, preparation is the key to success." This chapter elucidates the preoperative workup and exercises that can be done by patients to optimize early return of urinary continence and erectile function after surgery. Pelvic floor muscle training is a well-established program that should be instituted prior to surgery as numerous studies have shown improvement in continence rates postoperatively. Typically, it is easier for patients to incorporate these exercises after surgery when they have been introduced to them preoperatively. Also, the term "prehabilitation" or "prehab" has been introduced in the urologic literature. This encompasses everything from pelvic floor exercises for early return of continence to prophylactic PDE5 inhibitor use to augment erectile blood flow preoperatively and increase sensitivity to the medication after surgery. Prehab should be a standard part of preoperative counseling for patients undergoing radical prostatectomy.

References

1. American Cancer Society. Facts & figures 2022. Atlanta: American Cancer Society; 2022.
2. National Comprehensive Cancer Network. Prostate Cancer (Version 1.2023). January 15, 2023.
3. Moul JW. Radical prostatectomy versus radiation therapy for clinically localized prostate carcinoma: the butcher and the baker selling their wares. Cancer. 2002;95(2):211–4.
4. Halpern JA, et al. National trends in prostate biopsy and radical prostatectomy volumes following the US preventive services task force guidelines against prostate-specific antigen screening. JAMA Surg. 2017;152(2):192–8.
5. Walsh PC, Donker PJ. Impotence following radical prostatectomy: insight into etiology and prevention. J Urol. 1982;128(3):492–7.
6. Groutz A, et al. The pathophysiology of post-radical prostatectomy incontinence: a clinical and video urodynamic study. J Urol. 2000;163(6):1767–70.
7. Matsukawa Y, et al. De novo overactive bladder after robot-assisted laparoscopic radical prostatectomy. Neurourol Urodyn. 2018;37(6):2008–14.
8. Hosier GW, et al. Overactive bladder and storage lower urinary tract symptoms following radical prostatectomy. Urology. 2016;94:193–7.
9. Kielb SJ, Clemens JQ. Comprehensive urodynamics evaluation of 146 men with incontinence after radical prostatectomy. Urology. 2005;66(2):392–6.
10. Wang R, et al. Risk factors and quality of life for post-prostatectomy vesicourethral anastomotic stenoses. Urology. 2012;79(2):449–57.
11. Webb DR, Sethi K, Gee K. An analysis of the causes of bladder neck contracture after open and robot-assisted laparoscopic radical prostatectomy. BJU Int. 2009;103(7):957–63.
12. Breyer BN, et al. Incidence of bladder neck contracture after robot-assisted laparoscopic and open radical prostatectomy. BJU Int. 2010;106(11):1734–8.
13. Park R, et al. Anastomotic strictures following radical prostatectomy: insights into incidence, effectiveness of intervention, effect on continence, and factors predisposing to occurrence. Urology. 2001;57(4):742–6.
14. Silva LA, et al. Surgery for stress urinary incontinence due to presumed sphincter deficiency after prostate surgery. Cochrane Database Syst Rev. 2014;2014(9):CD008306.
15. N.N.I.f.H.a.C. Excellence Lower urinary tract symptoms in men: management. 2010.
16. Trofimenko V, Myers JB, Brant WO. Post-prostatectomy incontinence: how common and bothersome is it really? Sex Med Rev. 2017;5(4):536–43.

17. Desautel MG, Kapoor R, Badlani GH. Sphincteric incontinence: the primary cause of post-prostatectomy incontinence in patients with prostate cancer. Neurourol Urodyn. 1997;16(3):153–60.
18. Gudziak MR, McGuire EJ, Gormley EA. Urodynamic assessment of urethral sphincter function in post-prostatectomy incontinence. J Urol. 1996;156(3):1131–4; discussion 1134–5
19. Chao R, Mayo ME. Incontinence after radical prostatectomy: detrusor or sphincter causes. J Urol. 1995;154(1):16–8.
20. Dubbelman YD, Bosch JL. Urethral sphincter function before and after radical prostatectomy: systematic review of the prognostic value of various assessment techniques. Neurourol Urodyn. 2013;32(7):957–63.
21. Gerullis H, et al. Sphincter lesions after radical prostatectomy-evaluation and classification. J Endourol. 2011;25(6):1075–80.
22. Holm HV, et al. Severe postprostatectomy incontinence: is there an association between preoperative urodynamic findings and outcome of incontinence surgery? Scand J Urol. 2015;49(3):250–9.
23. Aanestad O, et al. Interference pattern in the urethral sphincter: a quantitative electromyographic study in patients before and after radical retropubic prostatectomy. Scand J Urol Nephrol. 1998;32(6):378–82.
24. Liu S, et al. Sphincter electromyography in patients after radical prostatectomy and cystoprostatectomy. Br J Urol. 1992;69(4):397–403.
25. Burnett AL, Mostwin JL. In situ anatomical study of the male urethral sphincteric complex: relevance to continence preservation following major pelvic surgery. J Urol. 1998;160(4):1301–6.
26. Myers RP, et al. Anatomy of radical prostatectomy as defined by magnetic resonance imaging. J Urol. 1998;159(6):2148–58.
27. Strasser H, et al. Transurethral ultrasound: evaluation of anatomy and function of the rhabdosphincter of the male urethra. J Urol. 1998;159(1):100–4; discussion 104–5
28. Mendoza PJ, et al. Pelvic anatomy on preoperative magnetic resonance imaging can predict early continence after robot-assisted radical prostatectomy. J Endourol. 2011;25(1):51–5.
29. Nguyen L, Jhaveri J, Tewari A. Surgical technique to overcome anatomical shortcoming: balancing post-prostatectomy continence outcomes of urethral sphincter lengths on preoperative magnetic resonance imaging. J Urol. 2008;179(5):1907–11.
30. Coakley FV, et al. Urinary continence after radical retropubic prostatectomy: relationship with membranous urethral length on preoperative endorectal magnetic resonance imaging. J Urol. 2002;168(3):1032–5.
31. Paparel P, et al. Recovery of urinary continence after radical prostatectomy: association with urethral length and urethral fibrosis measured by preoperative and postoperative endorectal magnetic resonance imaging. Eur Urol. 2009;55(3):629–37.
32. Minervini R, et al. Urodynamic evaluation of urinary incontinence following radical prostatectomy: our experience. Acta Urol Belg. 1996;64(4):5–8.
33. Kleinhans B, et al. Changes of urodynamic findings after radical retropubic prostatectomy. Eur Urol. 1999;35(3):217–21; discussion 221–2
34. Dubbelman YD, et al. Urodynamic quantification of decrease in sphincter function after radical prostatectomy: relation to postoperative continence status and the effect of intensive pelvic floor muscle exercises. Neurourol Urodyn. 2012;31(5):646–51.
35. Hammerer P, Huland H. Urodynamic evaluation of changes in urinary control after radical retropubic prostatectomy. J Urol. 1997;157(1):233–6.
36. Majoros A, et al. Urinary incontinence and voiding dysfunction after radical retropubic prostatectomy (prospective urodynamic study). Neurourol Urodyn. 2006;25(1):2–7.
37. Song C, et al. Urodynamic interpretation of changing bladder function and voiding pattern after radical prostatectomy: a long-term follow-up. BJU Int. 2010;106(5):681–6.
38. Pfister C, et al. Assessment of the intrinsic urethral sphincter component function in postprostatectomy urinary incontinence. Neurourol Urodyn. 2002;21(3):194–7.

39. Rudy DC, Woodside JR, Crawford ED. Urodynamic evaluation of incontinence in patients undergoing modified Campbell radical retropubic prostatectomy: a prospective study. J Urol. 1984;132(4):708–12.
40. John H, et al. Effect of radical prostatectomy on sensory threshold and pressure transmission. J Urol. 2000;163(6):1761–6.
41. Eastham JA, et al. Risk factors for urinary incontinence after radical prostatectomy. J Urol. 1996;156(5):1707–13.
42. Bauer RM, et al. Contemporary management of postprostatectomy incontinence. Eur Urol. 2011;59(6):985–96.
43. Radomski SB. Practical evaluation of post-prostatectomy incontinence. Can Urol Assoc J. 2013;7(9–10 Suppl 4):S186–8.
44. Radomski SB, Herschorn S. Risk factors associated with penile prosthesis infection. J Urol. 1992;147(2):383–5.
45. Patel MI, et al. Preoperative pelvic floor physiotherapy improves continence after radical retropubic prostatectomy. Int J Urol. 2013;20(10):986–92.
46. Centemero A, et al. Preoperative pelvic floor muscle exercise for early continence after radical prostatectomy: a randomised controlled study. Eur Urol. 2010;57(6):1039–43.
47. Geraerts I, et al. Pelvic floor muscle training for erectile dysfunction and climacturia 1 year after nerve sparing radical prostatectomy: a randomized controlled trial. Int J Impot Res. 2016;28(1):9–13.
48. Burgio KL, et al. Preoperative biofeedback assisted behavioral training to decrease post-prostatectomy incontinence: a randomized, controlled trial. J Urol. 2006;175(1):196–201; discussion 201
49. Bales GT, et al. Effect of preoperative biofeedback/pelvic floor training on continence in men undergoing radical prostatectomy. Urology. 2000;56(4):627–30.
50. Manassero F, et al. Contribution of early intensive prolonged pelvic floor exercises on urinary continence recovery after bladder neck-sparing radical prostatectomy: results of a prospective controlled randomized trial. Neurourol Urodyn. 2007;26(7):985–9.
51. Tal R, et al. Erectile function recovery rate after radical prostatectomy: a meta-analysis. J Sex Med. 2009;6(9):2538–46.
52. Magheli A, Burnett AL. Erectile dysfunction following prostatectomy: prevention and treatment. Nat Rev Urol. 2009;6(8):415–27.
53. Takenaka A, et al. Variation in course of cavernous nerve with special reference to details of topographic relationships near prostatic apex: histologic study using male cadavers. Urology. 2005;65(1):136–42.
54. Stanford JL, et al. Urinary and sexual function after radical prostatectomy for clinically localized prostate cancer: the Prostate Cancer Outcomes Study. JAMA. 2000;283(3):354–60.
55. Patel VR, et al. Periurethral suspension stitch during robot-assisted laparoscopic radical prostatectomy: description of the technique and continence outcomes. Eur Urol. 2009;56(3):472–8.
56. Dalela D, et al. A pragmatic randomized controlled trial examining the impact of the Retzius-sparing approach on early urinary continence recovery after robot-assisted radical prostatectomy. Eur Urol. 2017;72(5):677–85.
57. Briganti A, Montorsi F. Penile rehabilitation after radical prostatectomy. Nat Clin Pract Urol. 2006;3(8):400–1.
58. Sari Motlagh R, et al. Penile rehabilitation strategy after nerve sparing radical prostatectomy: a systematic review and network meta-analysis of randomized trials. J Urol. 2021;205(4):1018–30.
59. Mulhall J, et al. The use of an erectogenic pharmacotherapy regimen following radical prostatectomy improves recovery of spontaneous erectile function. J Sex Med. 2005;2(4):532–40; discussion 540–2
60. Albersen M, et al. Preclinical evidence for the benefits of penile rehabilitation therapy following nerve-sparing radical prostatectomy. Adv Urol. 2008;2008:594868.

61. Baccaglini W, et al. The role of the low-intensity extracorporeal shockwave therapy on penile rehabilitation after radical prostatectomy: a randomized clinical trial. J Sex Med. 2020;17(4):688–94.
62. Ficarra V, et al. Systematic review and meta-analysis of studies reporting potency rates after robot-assisted radical prostatectomy. Eur Urol. 2012;62(3):418–30.
63. Hanno PM, Wein AJ, Malkowicz SB. Penn clinical manual of urology. Philadelphia: Saunders/Elsevier; 2007. xx, 986 p.
64. Althof SE, et al. Sildenafil citrate improves self-esteem, confidence, and relationships in men with erectile dysfunction: results from an international, multi-center, double-blind, placebo-controlled trial. J Sex Med. 2006;3(3):521–9.
65. Abdo CH. The male sexual quotient: a brief, self-administered questionnaire to assess male sexual satisfaction. J Sex Med. 2007;4(2):382–9.
66. Ramanathan R, et al. Predictive correlation between the International Index of Erectile Function (IIEF) and Sexual Health Inventory for Men (SHIM): implications for calculating a derived SHIM for clinical use. J Sex Med. 2007;4(5):1336–44.
67. Bach P, et al. Quality of life of patients after retropubic prostatectomy – pre- and postoperative scores of the EORTC QLQ-C30 and QLQ-PR25. Health Qual Life Outcomes. 2011;9:93.
68. Leufgens F, et al. Quality of life changes >10 years after postoperative radiation therapy after radical prostatectomy for prostate cancer. Int J Radiat Oncol Biol Phys. 2019;105(2):382–8.

Technical Innovations to Optimize Early Return of Urinary Continence

4

Adriana M. Pedraza, Raghav Gupta, Dhruti Patel, Vinayak Wagaskar, Manish Choudhary, and Ash Tewari

Preservation of Periprostatic Structures

Bladder Neck

The region at the outlet of the urinary bladder and the point of entry to the prostatic urethra is commonly referred to as the bladder neck. This area is formed by a combination of structures, including the detrusor muscle, the vesical sphincter (musculus sphincter vesicae), and the prostatic tissue located in close proximity [1]. The significance of bladder neck preservation during robotic-assisted radical prostatectomy (RARP) remains a controversial topic, as studies have presented conflicting results [2–6]. However, a single-blind, randomized controlled trial showed that preserving the bladder neck resulted in higher rates of urinary continence without compromising surgical margins. The authors suggested that the preservation of sensory nerve fibers could be responsible for this improvement by maintaining feedback to the micturition center and optimizing its interaction with the external urethral sphincter [7]. Similarly, Sood et al. conducted a study to examine the impact of different techniques on early continence following RARP. Of note, transvesical approaches that maintained the Retzius space but did not spare the bladder neck had the poorest continence outcomes. Conversely, techniques that preserved the bladder neck, with or without the Retzius space, resulted in the fastest recovery of urinary continence. Furthermore, bladder neck preservation was the sole independent

Supplementary Information The online version contains supplementary material available at https://doi.org/10.1007/978-3-031-64245-6_4.

A. M. Pedraza (✉) · R. Gupta · D. Patel · V. Wagaskar · M. Choudhary · A. Tewari
Department of Urology, Icahn School of Medicine at Mount Sinai, New York City, NY, USA
e-mail: Raghav.gupta@mountsinai.org; Dhruti.patel@mountsinai.org; Manish.Choudhary@mountsinai.org; Ash.tewari@mountsinai.org

S. Razdan, S. Razdan (eds.), *Urinary Continence and Sexual Function After Robotic Prostatectomy, Radiation, and Novel Therapies*,
https://doi.org/10.1007/978-3-031-64245-6_4

predictor of continence recovery at both 1 week and 1 month after surgery [8]. On the other hand, preservation techniques have been found to result in lower incidences of bladder neck contracture, which may also play a role in the enhancement of early continence [9]. These findings suggest that the preservation of the bladder neck could be a crucial factor in achieving better outcomes in urinary continence for patients undergoing RARP. However, in cases where the median lobe is particularly large, achieving this preservation may be challenging.

Neurovascular Bundles

The distribution of periprostatic nerves is intricate and extends beyond the typical posterolateral neurovascular bundles that Walsh and Donker originally described in 1982 [10]. Various authors have characterized this arrangement as a fanlike or hammock-like structure [11–13]. For instance, Tewari et al. suggested a trizonal hammock where the inferior hypogastric plexus (IHP) represented the proximal neural plate (PNP), and the nerves encircling the prostate were referred to as the predominant neurovascular bundle (PNB) and accessory neural pathways (ANP) as shown in Fig. 4.1 [13].

While it was traditionally believed that the external urethral sphincter (EUS) was innervated exclusively by somatic nerve fibers, and the internal urethral sphincter (IUS) by autonomic nerves, Nyangoh Timoh et al. challenged this notion through detailed fetal anatomic studies. They found that the EUS also receives innervation from parasympathetic fibers. Additionally, the authors described that autonomic and somatic fibers from the pudendal nerve communicate within the levator ani muscle. The autonomic nerves from the IHP, mainly lateroprostatic and prerectal fibers, innervate both the IUS and EUS. Some of those autonomic fibers run along the posterolateral neurovascular bundles, while others traverse from the IHP to the posteromedial region of the prostate apex, above and through the rectourethral muscle [14]. Bessede et al. conducted a thorough review that highlighted the complex innervation of the sphincter, with contributions from both the somatic and

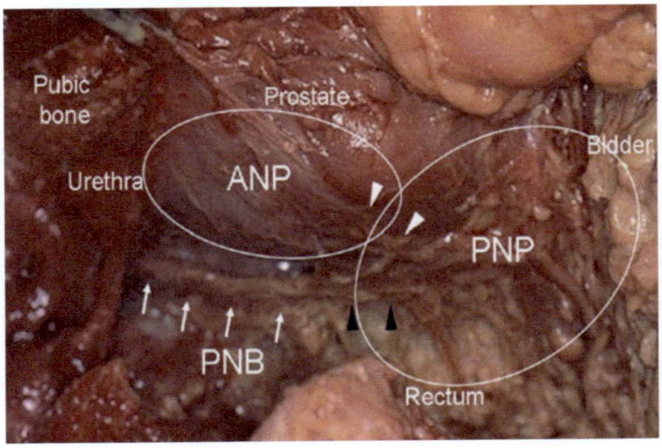

Fig. 4.1 Trilevel neural zone concept. Lateral view from the left side after the removal of the pubic bone. Black arrowheads indicate the continuity of PNP and PNB (arrows), and white arrowheads indicate the continuity of PNP and ANP. Fresh cadaver dissection. (Reprinted with permission from Tewari et al. [13])

autonomic nervous systems. As explained by the authors, the neuroanatomy of the US involves significant cross-communication, redundancy, and potentially neuroplasticity [15]. The aforementioned indicates that sparing the "neural hammock" is essential for maintaining both urinary continence and erectile function. In fact, Srivastava et al. [16] showed that patients who underwent a more aggressive nerve-sparing approach, based on the grading system proposed by Tewari et al. [17], (Fig. 4.2) experienced earlier return of urinary continence. Similarly, Suardi et al. investigated a group of 1249 patients who had undergone radical prostatectomy and observed that the nerve-sparing status was a significant factor in predicting the recovery of urinary continence ($P = 0.002$). Furthermore, patients who received bilateral nerve sparing had a 1.8-fold higher chance of achieving full urinary continence recovery ($P < 0.001$) compared to other groups.

Anterior Periprostatic Structures

The detrusor apron, first described by Santorini in 1724, is an extension of the longitudinal smooth muscle that stretches beyond the bladder neck and into the pubovesical muscle [18]. It is accompanied by a vascular plexus, and together they constitute the "pubovesical complex." In the past, these structures were typically bunched in the midline and sectioned to enhance visibility and hemostasis during surgery. However, contemporary approaches prioritize their preservation, a revolutionary concept introduced by Galfano et al. in 2010 through the Retzius-Sparing Robot-Assisted Laparoscopic Prostatectomy (RS-RALP), also known as Bocciardi's technique [19]. RS-RALP focuses on preserving the anterior periprostatic tissue, including the detrusor apron, Santorini plexus, puboprostatic ligaments, endopelvic fascia, and accessory pudendal arteries. It has been found to result in a faster functional recovery, with immediate continence rates of 70–76%, as compared to 21–60% with the standard RALP. However, there is an ongoing debate regarding its impact on positive surgical margin rates, with some studies indicating no

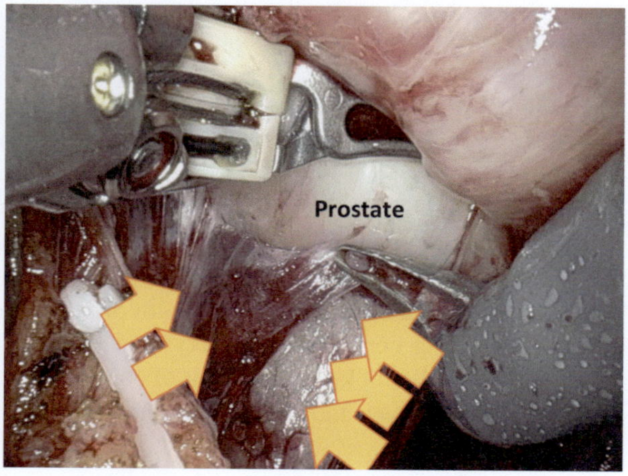

Fig. 4.2 Grade 1 nerve-sparing (maximal nerve preservation). The yellow arrows show the PNB

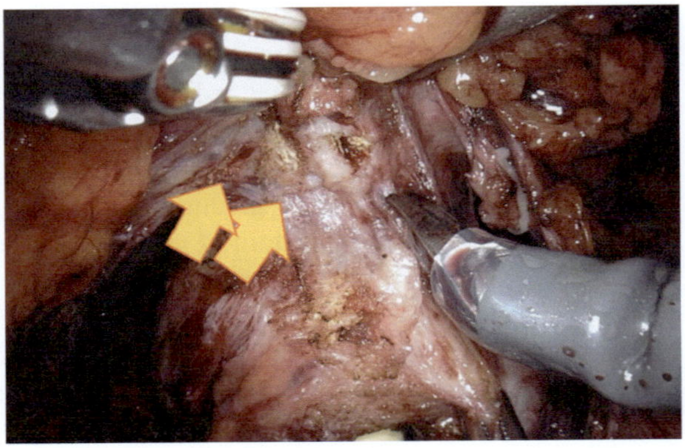

Fig. 4.3 The "hood technique" for preserving the anterior periprostatic structures. The yellow arrows indicate the location of the hood

differences [20, 21] and others suggesting higher rates [22]. Tewari and colleagues developed an alternative method, the "hood technique" (Fig. 4.3.), grounded on the same fundamental principle. This approach achieved continence rates of 83% 4 weeks after surgery [23]. In addition, it offers the ability to tailor nerve sparing to individual patients, simplifies the management of significant median lobes, and allows the visualization of ureteral orifices, enabling the placement of stents if needed and minimizing the risk of ureteral injuries. Elsayed et al. also provided support for these findings. This group found that patients who received modified RALP, in which the endopelvic fascia, puboprostatic ligaments, and dorsal venous complex were spared, and hydrodissection of the neurovascular bundles was carried out, had earlier urinary continence at 4 weeks, 3 months, and 6 months, with a median time to social continence of 1.9 months compared to 5.4 months for those who did not receive this modified surgery [24]. An advantage of anterior approaches, such as the hood and the latter technique, is that urologists are already acquainted with the involved anatomical landmarks. This familiarity improves their versatility and reproducibility (Video 4.1).

Maximal Urethral Length

The segment of the urethra known as the membranous runs between the prostatic and bulbar urethra, spanning from the apex of the prostate as it passes through the urogenital diaphragm (Fig. 4.4). Preserving the longitudinally oriented smooth muscle layer of the membranous urethra has been demonstrated to have an impact on continence outcomes. In their systematic review and meta-analysis, Mungovan et al. evaluated four studies with more than 1700 patients. They found a significant correlation between the preoperative length of membranous urethra and the probability of achieving continence recovery. Specifically, they observed that for each additional millimeter of length, the odds of continence recovery increased by 5–15% [25]. Likewise, Nguyen and colleagues conducted an evaluation on the significance

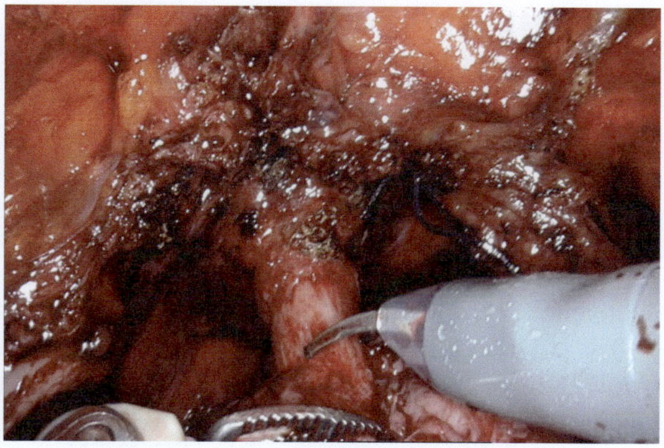

Fig. 4.4 Maximum urethral length preserved

of preserving maximal urethral length (MUL) in relation to continence rates. Their findings revealed that patients with a MUL ≥ 14 mm had better continence rates. However, for those with a MUL shorter than 14 mm, implementing additional techniques such as total anatomic reconstruction helped to decrease the gap in outcomes compared to those with longer urethras [26].

The use of preoperative multiparametric magnetic resonance imaging (mpMRI) has led to a greater emphasis on assessing not only the membranous urethral length but also the shape of the prostate apex as 10–40% of the functional urethra is covered by its parenchyma [27]. Lee et al. reported that patients with a type D prostatic apex, which does not overlap the membranous urethra either anteriorly or posteriorly, experienced significantly earlier return of continence [28].

There have been several techniques developed for MUL preservation, and among them is the one introduced by Schlomm and colleagues [27], which involved preserving the portion of the urethral sphincter located within the prostate. This technique yielded superior early continence results, without any significant differences in long-term continence outcomes.

In order to preserve the MUL during surgery, it is important to be aware of the surgical margins. To address this issue, Tewari and colleagues developed a technique that involved a synchronous urethral transection through a retro-apical approach. This technique significantly improved the visualization of the membranous urethral boundaries, leading to a lower incidence of positive surgical margins (1.4% vs 4.4%, $P = 0.04$) [29]. The collar technique has also focused on this matter. Bianchi and colleagues described this approach [30], which involves an incision of the urethral sphincter complex 2–3 mm distally to the apex. The underlying smooth muscle is then exposed and incised closer to the apex, preserving the maximum length of the lissosphincter. This method has proven effective in decreasing positive surgical margins during radical prostatectomy. Both these techniques highlight the importance of striking a balance between preserving the MUL and maintaining oncologic outcomes during robotic-assisted radical prostatectomy.

Total Anatomical Reconstruction

Rocco first introduced the principles of reconstruction, wherein he described the restoration of the posterior aspect of the rhabdosphincter and its effect on the time to achieve continence after a radical retropubic prostatectomy [31, 32]. Over time, modifications have been proposed, culminating in the development of the total anatomical reconstruction (TAR) technique. This innovative approach has been shown by various studies to yield promising results in terms of earlier recovery of urinary continence [31, 33–35].

The TAR technique entails a comprehensive posterior reconstruction, which involves the reattachment of Denonvilliers' fascia and the retrotrigonal layer to the median raphe, along with the attachment of the bladder neck (excluding the bladder mucosa) to the posterior aspect of the rhabdosphincter (Fig. 4.5.). The TAR procedure also involves the performance of the urethrovesical anastomosis (Fig. 4.6), followed by the anterior reconstruction. During the anterior reconstruction phase, the surgeon meticulously approaches the muscular fibers of the bladder and the previously dissected periurethral tissue. Moreover, the endopelvic fascia and puboprostatic ligaments are reattached to the detrusor apron in cases where the anterior structures were not preserved [36].

The study conducted by Manfredi et al. demonstrated notable outcomes of the TAR technique, as they reported continence rates of 59%, 80%, and 95% at 1 week, 4 weeks, and 12 months post-surgery, respectively. In a randomized controlled trial conducted by Menon et al., it was found that higher rates of urinary continence were achieved when periprostatic tissues were reconstructed, particularly in cases where a double-layer urethrovesical anastomosis was performed [37]. On the other hand, Tewari et al. described the augmentation of the TAR technique that involved the incorporation of dynamic detrusor cuff trigonoplasty. The authors observed that the addition of this technique led to continence rates of 65% within just 2 weeks following surgery [35]. Similarly, Zanoni et al. investigated the use of the TAR technique combined with a sling using the retrotrigonal muscular layer and observed favorable

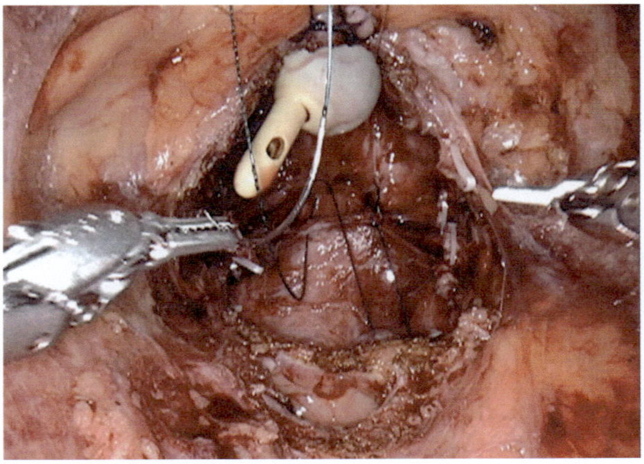

Fig. 4.5 Posterior reconstruction

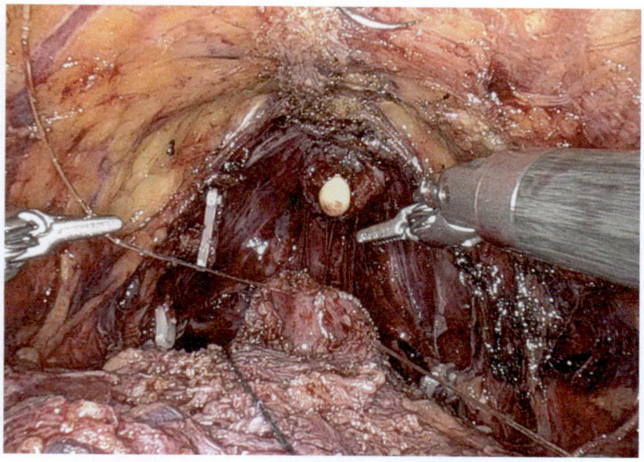

Fig. 4.6 Watertight urethrovesical anastomosis

outcomes. The authors found that the combined technique yielded continence rates as high as 72% in 1 week following surgery. These findings suggest that the TAR, either alone or in combination with other approaches, can be effective in promoting urinary continence recovery [38].

In summary, achieving optimal urinary continence recovery after prostate surgery requires attention to several factors. These include thorough preoperative assessment and planning, preservation of periprostatic structures whenever possible, and meticulous reconstruction as needed. Surgeons must be mindful of the neural anatomy to avoid injury, particularly during the apical dissection phase where multiple structures converge. Careful dissection is fundamental to achieve the desired outcomes. Ultimately, the aim is to restore the anatomy as closely as possible to its pre-surgical state, whether through preservation or reconstruction of the relevant structures.

Take-Home Message

We published our work on maximal urethral length preservation (MULP) technique in 2014. Since that time, there have been numerous descriptions of methods to maintain continence focused on lengthening perceived and actual membranous urethral length, reconstructing the anterior prostatic suspensory attachments, and preserving the levator muscle complex and neurovascular hammock. Fundamentally, urinary continence after prostate surgery requires an interplay of intrinsic sphincter/bladder neck preservation, as well as support from deep pelvic structures that contribute to continence in an accessory fashion.

References

1. Walz J, Epstein JI, Ganzer R, et al. A critical analysis of the current knowledge of surgical anatomy of the prostate related to optimisation of cancer control and preservation of continence and erection in candidates for radical prostatectomy: an update. Eur Urol. 2016;70(2):301–11. https://doi.org/10.1016/j.eururo.2016.01.026.

2. Pedraza AM, Wagaskar V, Parekh S, Tewari A. Technical advances in nerve-sparing and continence preservation. Curr Opin Urol. 2022;32(2):204–10. https://doi.org/10.1097/MOU.0000000000000958.
3. Gomez CA, Soloway MS, Civantos F, Hachiya T. Bladder neck preservation and its impact on positive surgical margins during radical prostatectomy. Urology. 1993;42(6):689–93. https://doi.org/10.1016/0090-4295(93)90534-H.
4. Deliveliotis C, Protogerou V, Alargof E, Varkarakis J. Radical prostatectomy: bladder neck preservation and puboprostatic ligament sparing – effects on continence and positive margins. Urology. 2002;60(5):855–8. https://doi.org/10.1016/S0090-4295(02)01956-8.
5. Nyarangi-Dix JN, Tichy D, Hatiboglu G, Pahernik S, Tosev G, Hohenfellner M. Complete bladder neck preservation promotes long-term post-prostatectomy continence without compromising midterm oncological outcome: analysis of a randomised controlled cohort. World J Urol. 2018;36(3):349–55. https://doi.org/10.1007/s00345-017-2134-1.
6. Licht MR, Klein EA, Tuason L, Levin H. Impact of bladder neck preservation during radical prostatectomy on continence and cancer control. Urology. 1994;44(6):883–7. https://doi.org/10.1016/S0090-4295(94)80175-4.
7. Nyarangi-Dix JN, Radtke JP, Hadaschik B, Pahernik S, Hohenfellner M. Impact of complete bladder neck preservation on urinary continence, quality of life and surgical margins after radical prostatectomy: a randomized, controlled, single blind trial. J Urol. 2013;189(3):891–8. https://doi.org/10.1016/j.juro.2012.09.082.
8. Sood A, Grauer R, Jeong W, et al. Evaluating post radical prostatectomy mechanisms of early continence. Prostate. 2022;82:1186–95. https://doi.org/10.1002/pros.24371.
9. Shelfo SW, Obek C, Soloway MS. Update on bladder neck preservation during radical retropubic prostatectomy: impact on pathologic outcome, anastomotic strictures, and continence. Urology 1998;51(1):73–78.
10. Walsh PC, Donker PJ. Impotence following radical prostatectomy: insight into etiology and prevention. J Urol. 1982;128(3):492–7. https://doi.org/10.1016/S0022-5347(17)53012-8.
11. Costello AJ, Dowdle BW, Namdarian B, Pedersen J, Murphy DG. Immunohistochemical study of the cavernous nerves in the periprostatic region. BJU Int. 2011;107(8):1210–5. https://doi.org/10.1111/j.1464-410X.2010.09711.x.
12. Costello AJ, Brooks M, Cole OJ. Anatomical studies of the neurovascular bundle and cavernosal nerves. BJU Int. 2004;94(7):1071–6. https://doi.org/10.1111/j.1464-410X.2004.05106.x.
13. Tewari A, Takenaka A, Mtui E, et al. The proximal neurovascular plate and the tri-zonal neural architecture around the prostate gland: importance in the athermal robotic technique of nerve-sparing prostatectomy. BJU Int. 2006;98(2):314–23. https://doi.org/10.1111/j.1464-410X.2006.06266.x.
14. Nyangoh Timoh K, Moszkowicz D, Creze M, et al. The male external urethral sphincter is autonomically innervated. Clin Anat. 2021;34(2):263–71. https://doi.org/10.1002/ca.23698.
15. Bessede T, Sooriakumaran P, Takenaka A, Tewari A. Neural supply of the male urethral sphincter: comprehensive anatomical review and implications for continence recovery after radical prostatectomy. World J Urol. 2017;35(4):549–65. https://doi.org/10.1007/s00345-016-1901-8.
16. Srivastava A, Chopra S, Pham A, et al. Effect of a risk-stratified grade of nerve-sparing technique on early return of continence after robot-assisted laparoscopic radical prostatectomy. Eur Urol. 2013;63(3):438–44. https://doi.org/10.1016/j.eururo.2012.07.009.
17. Tewari AK, Srivastava A, Huang MW, et al. Anatomical grades of nerve sparing: a risk-stratified approach to neural-hammock sparing during robot-assisted radical prostatectomy (RARP). BJU Int. 2011;108(6 B):984–92. https://doi.org/10.1111/j.1464-410X.2011.10565.x.
18. Myers RP. Avascular plane: relevance to radical Retropubic prostatectomy—anatomic and surgical commentary. Urology. 2002;4295(02):472–9.
19. Galfano A, Ascione A, Grimaldi S, Petralia G, Strada E, Bocciardi AM. A new anatomic approach for robot-assisted laparoscopic prostatectomy: a feasibility study for completely intrafascial surgery. Eur Urol. 2010;58(3):457–61. https://doi.org/10.1016/j.eururo.2010.06.008.

20. Umari P, Eden C, Cahill D, Rizzo M, Eden D, Sooriakumaran P. Retzius-sparing versus standard robot-assisted radical prostatectomy: a comparative prospective study of nearly 500 patients. J Urol. 2021;205(3):780–90. https://doi.org/10.1097/JU.0000000000001435.
21. Liu J, Zhang J, Yang Z, et al. Comparison of Retzius-sparing and conventional robot-assisted laparoscopic radical prostatectomy regarding continence and sexual function: an updated meta-analysis. Prostate Cancer Prostatic Dis. 2021;(June):1–8. https://doi.org/10.1038/s41391-021-00459-5.
22. Checcucci E, Veccia A, Fiori C, et al. Retzius-sparing robot-assisted radical prostatectomy vs the standard approach: a systematic review and analysis of comparative outcomes. BJU Int. 2020;125(1):8–16. https://doi.org/10.1111/bju.14887.
23. Wagaskar VG, Mittal A, Sobotka S, et al. Hood technique for robotic radical prostatectomy—preserving Periurethral anatomical structures in the space of Retzius and sparing the pouch of Douglas, enabling early return of continence without compromising surgical margin rates. Eur Urol. 2021;80(2):213–21. https://doi.org/10.1016/j.eururo.2020.09.044.
24. Elsayed AS, Ely HB, Abdelhakim MA, et al. Preservation of endopelvic fascia, puboprostatic ligaments, dorsal venous complex and hydrodissection of the neurovascular bundles during robot-assisted radical prostatectomy: a video demonstration and propensity score matched outcomes. Urol Video J. 2022;14:100143. https://doi.org/10.1016/j.urolvj.2022.100143.
25. Mungovan SF, Sandhu JS, Akin O, Smart NA, Graham PL, Patel MI. Preoperative membranous urethral length measurement and continence recovery following radical prostatectomy: a systematic review and meta-analysis. Eur Urol. 2017;71(3):368–78. https://doi.org/10.1016/j.eururo.2016.06.023.
26. Nguyen L, Jhaveri J, Tewari A. Surgical technique to overcome anatomical shortcoming: balancing post-prostatectomy continence outcomes of urethral sphincter lengths on preoperative magnetic resonance imaging. J Urol. 2008;179(5):1907–11. https://doi.org/10.1016/j.juro.2008.01.036.
27. Schlomm T, Heinzer H, Steuber T, et al. Full functional-length urethral sphincter preservation during radical prostatectomy. Eur Urol. 2011;60(2):320–9. https://doi.org/10.1016/j.eururo.2011.02.040.
28. Lee SE, Byun SS, Lee HJ, et al. Impact of variations in prostatic apex shape on early recovery of urinary continence after radical retropubic prostatectomy. Urology. 2006;68(1):137–41. https://doi.org/10.1016/j.urology.2006.01.021.
29. Tewari AK, Srivastava A, Mudaliar K, et al. Anatomical retro-apical technique of synchronous (posterior and anterior) urethral transection: a novel approach for ameliorating apical margin positivity during robotic radical prostatectomy. BJU Int. 2010;106(9):1364–73. https://doi.org/10.1111/j.1464-410X.2010.09318.x.
30. Bianchi L, Turri FM, Larcher A, et al. A novel approach for apical dissection during robot-assisted radical prostatectomy: the "collar" technique. Eur Urol Focus. 2018;4(5):677–85. https://doi.org/10.1016/j.euf.2018.01.004.
31. Rocco F, Carmignani L, Acquati P, et al. Restoration of posterior aspect of rhabdosphincter shortens continence time after radical retropubic prostatectomy. J Urol. 2006;175(6):2201–6. https://doi.org/10.1016/S0022-5347(06)00262-X.
32. Rocco F, Carmignani L, Acquati P, et al. Early continence recovery after open radical prostatectomy with restoration of the posterior aspect of the rhabdosphincter. Eur Urol. 2007;52(2):376–83. https://doi.org/10.1016/j.eururo.2007.01.109.
33. Tewari A, Jhaveri J, Rao S, et al. Total reconstruction of the vesico-urethral junction. BJU Int. 2008;101(7):871–7. https://doi.org/10.1111/j.1464-410X.2008.07424.x.
34. Porpiglia F, Bertolo R, Manfredi M, et al. Total anatomical reconstruction during robot-assisted radical prostatectomy: implications on early recovery of urinary continence. Eur Urol. 2016;69(3):485–95. https://doi.org/10.1016/j.eururo.2015.08.005.
35. Tewari AK, Ali A, Ghareeb G, et al. Improving time to continence after robot-assisted laparoscopic prostatectomy: augmentation of the total anatomic reconstruction technique by adding dynamic detrusor cuff trigonoplasty and suprapubic tube placement. J Endourol. 2012;26(12):1546–52. https://doi.org/10.1089/end.2012.0544.

36. Manfredi M, Checcucci E, Fiori C, et al. Total anatomical reconstruction during robot-assisted radical prostatectomy: focus on urinary continence recovery and related complications after 1000 procedures. BJU Int. 2019;124(3):477–86. https://doi.org/10.1111/bju.14716.
37. Menon M, Muhletaler F, Campos M, Peabody JO. Assessment of early continence after reconstruction of the periprostatic tissues in patients undergoing computer assisted (robotic) prostatectomy: results of a 2 group parallel randomized controlled trial. J Urol. 2008;180(3):1018–23. https://doi.org/10.1016/j.juro.2008.05.046.
38. Zanoni ML, Grizzi F, Maffei D, et al. Retrotrigonal muscular layer sling associated with total anatomical reconstruction in robot-assisted radical prostatectomy and early continence. World J Urol. 2021;39(7):2475–81. https://doi.org/10.1007/s00345-020-03500-9.

Technical Innovations to Optimize Early Return of Erectile Function After Radical Prostatectomy

5

Shirin Razdan, Sneha Parekh, and Sanjay Razdan

Introduction

Robotic assisted laparoscopic prostatectomy (RALP) has been well documented for its PENTAFECTA outcomes of oncologic control, lower transfusion rates, less incontinence, fewer positive surgical margins (PSM), and improved potency. To achieve this goal, understanding the anatomy and visualizing key landmarks in real time to perform athermal, traction-free nerve sparing (NS) using newer optimization techniques is needed.

Supplementary Information The online version contains supplementary material available at https://doi.org/10.1007/978-3-031-64245-6_5.

S. Razdan
Miami Robotic Surgery at the Comprehensive Urologic Surgery Institute, Miami, FL, USA

S. Parekh
Larkin Palm Springs Hospital, Hialeah, FL, USA

S. Razdan (✉)
International Robotic Institute for Prostate Cancer, Miami, FL, USA

S. Razdan, S. Razdan (eds.), *Urinary Continence and Sexual Function After Robotic Prostatectomy, Radiation, and Novel Therapies*,
https://doi.org/10.1007/978-3-031-64245-6_5

The initial description of the neurovascular bundle (NVB) anatomy was by Walsh and Donker [1], followed by further detailed 3D anatomic visualization in cadavers [2]. The intraoperative use of imaging and nerve stimulation studies has helped surgeon-scientists to redefine the cavernous nerve (CN) course while also aiding in improvement of the surgical technique for preservation of the prostate neuroanatomy and peri-prostatic architecture. While acceptable oncologic outcomes are always at the forefront, studies have demonstrated these new techniques and innovations give promising functional outcome results as well.

While the focus of this chapter is on intraoperative techniques to optimize erectile function after RALP, the urologist must keep in mind that penile rehabilitation using postoperative pharmacological, surgical, and regenerative therapies has also helped patients achieve early return of functional outcomes [3–11].

Anatomy of NVBs

The prostate and its surrounding structures, such as the seminal vesicles (SVs), peri-prostatic fascia, and urethra, are supplied by autonomic and somatic branches originating from the lower thoracolumbar (T11–L2) and sacral (S2–S4) vertebral centers. Nerve fibers from these centers coalesce to form the pelvic plexus, a plexus of nerves interposed with ganglion cells and fibro-fatty tissue. This was initially described by Walsh and Donker [1] as a fenestrated rectangular plate situated in the retroperitoneum laterally over the rectum in the sagittal plane. This proposed anatomy of the NVB and its projection to peri-prostatic structures have been supported by additional anatomical and clinical studies.

The pelvic plexus is denoted as the proximal neurovascular plate (PNP) by Tewari et al. [12] located lateral to the bladder neck, the SVs, and branches of the inferior vesical vessels. The autonomic fibers from the PNP are distributed into the NVB or predominant neurovascular bundle (PNB) and accessory neural pathway (ANP) in a spray-like pattern [13], with 60% of fibers on the posterolateral and 40% on the anterolateral prostate. The PNB is described as a tubular or cord-like structure that runs from the base to the apex posterolaterally within layers of the levator fascia. It varies in its course, shape, and size, thickest at the base and with maximal variability at the apex. It has ganglionic cells in close proximity or attachment to the prostate capsule; hence, careful athermal dissection of the capsule is needed to avoid damage to the ganglionic cells and preserve post-RALP functional outcome.

Course of NVB

Both the sympathetic and parasympathetic fibers in male fetuses run dorsolaterally toward the prostatic and membranous urethra and then pierce the urogenital diaphragm and supply the corpora cavernosa (CC) of the penis. As the prostate grows in adult males, it migrates ventrolaterally [14], forming a spray-like distribution of the NVB on the convex side of the prostate [12]. Further, the anterolateral nerves are a mix of parasympathetic (PNS) and sympathetic (SNS), traveling toward the prostatic stroma and other vascular structures such as the levator ani, SV, and rectum. In the mid-prostate, 18% of total PNS fibers are present in this anterolateral region and have no role in the pro-erectile innervation of penis, while the majority are located in the posterolateral surface [15]. These fibers converge again at the prostate apex, lying adjacent to the membranous urethra along the lateral and dorsolateral side of the urethra between the 3 and the 9 o'clock positions, sparing the dorsal median raphe. Hence, careful dorsal dissection at the prostatic apex and urethra, on the lateral prostate and SVs is important.

Cavernous Nerve (CN) and Its Variations

The CN is responsible for autonomic innervation to the penis and mediates penile erection [16].

The sympathetic and parasympathetic branches from T11 to 12 and S2 to S4, respectively, form the pelvic plexus. The two nerves branch out farther from the plexus and cross with each other to form the CN. The CN nerve interposes with the vessels of the NVB and traverse through the peri-prostatic fascial layers and pierce the rhabdosphincter, to reach the CC and the membranous urethra. The PNS nerve fibers supplying the corporal bodies and the membranous urethra further receive signals from the cerebral cortex. Various neurotransmitters such as neuronal nitric oxide synthase (nNOS) and endothelial NOS (eNOS) in the vascular and sinusoidal endothelium are released for erections.

Takenaka et al. [17] described the interindividual variation in the CN course near the rhabdosphincter and prostate apex, and a statistically significant difference was noted. This study showed that the CN pass through three sections: frontal, sagittal, and axial. The frontal and sagittal courses take place through a space between the levator ani and rhabdosphincter or via the levator fascia, on the lateral aspect of the prostate. This dorsoventral orientation changed from the apex to the urethra in the sagittal and axial plane from 7 to 8 o'clock position to the 10 to 11 o'clock position while remaining at 9 to 10 o'clock position in the frontal plane, giving some twigs ending in the sphincter area. In the axial plane, this nerve takes a tortuous course away from the prostate through the perirectal space, reaching the inferior level of the prostate apex. It gives branches to the rectourethralis at the dorsolateral side and finally innervating the urethra anterolaterally.

Alsaid et al. [17], in a detailed three-dimensional (3D) computer-assisted anatomic dissection, found that the anterior and anterolateral branches traverse through the undersurface of the venous complex and innervate the CC medially toward the penile hilum. In their study, the corpus spongiosum was supplied by the posterolateral extension of the NVB. The authors also demonstrated formation of CNs in the anterior and anterolateral prostate, specifically at the apex. Hence, the course and distribution of peri-prostatic nerves vary between individuals. Inclusion of intraoperative technologies such as multiphoton spectroscopy or fluoroscopy or 3D imaging and augmented reality models can aid urologists in visualizing these nerves in real time.

Peri-prostatic Fascia

The prostate is compactly surrounded by multilayered fascia, with the capsule surrounded by the visceral endopelvic fascia. Anteriorly, it is attached to the anterior fibromuscular stroma (AFMS), reaches the posterolateral prostate embracing the NVB medially, and becomes the pararectal fascia covering the rectum. Lateral to this layer is the fascia covering the levator ani muscle also known as the parietal endopelvic fascia [18]. These two layers at the lateral prostate border fuse and form a condensed line known as the arcus tendineus line. These form a landmark for fascial dissection during NS in RALP. These layers have intermingling vessels, nerves, fat, and connective tissue. Several studies have shown fascia-preserving surgical methods to give improved continence and EF results [3, 19].

Anatomic Landmarks for NS and Different Grading Systems of NS

Patel et al. [20] described five grades of NS based on the landmark artery of the peri-prostatic vasculature that runs on the lateral aspect of the prostate and medially to the NVB, known as the prostate or capsular artery. After dissecting the Denonvilliers fascia (DVF), and creating a plane toward the prostatic apex laterally, the pink prostate artery is noted. This grading system follows a retrograde approach of NS, with grade 5 being complete NS (>95%) at the pearly areolar tissue, grade 4 being nearly complete NS (75%) between the LA and prostatic capsule, grade 3 (50%) when the dissection plane is created at the lateral side of the artery after clipping the LA, grade 2 when several mm lateral to the LA and can be confirmed with intraoperative visualization of embedded arteries in the areolar tissue, and grade 1 (<50%) when there is a wide resection of the NVB (0% NS).

Tewari et al. [21] described the grades of NS based on the intraoperative examination of peri-prostatic fascial planes and venous distribution over the prostate. NS begins after sectioning the vas deferens and SV dissection with the posterior dissection of the prostate. When DVF is dissected completely, leaving all of its layers on the prostate, this is known as an extra-fascial dissection. When dissected partly between the anterior and posterior layers, it is known as inter-fascial dissection. Laterally, the LPF is encountered and four grades of NS are described. Grade 1 NS is the dissection between the prostatic capsule and LPF aka intrafascial dissection. Grade 2 is intrafascial dissection between the visceral and parietal layers of LPF. Grade 3 is dissection between the LPF and levator ani fascia, and grade 4 is dissecting all the fascial layers out. The author found better potency rates with grade 1 NS as compared to the incremental grades of NS [22].

Montorsi et al. [23] described four grades of the extent of NS, using the NVB as the landmark.

Stolzenburg et al. [24] used the peri-prostatic fascia as the landmark for the three grades of NS.

Preoperative Considerations

Briganti et al. [7] developed a model based on the extent of fascial preservation and postoperative erectile function (EF) after RALP. This model incorporates patient's age, preoperative international index of EF (IIEF) score, Charlson Comorbidity Index Score (CCSI), and use of clips for NS along with FP. It predicts postoperative IIEF-EF score.

The clinical utility and impact of MRI in the decision-making process for the extent of resection during radical prostatectomy (RP) has been well documented in a meta-analysis [25]. More recently, MRI-based 3D prostate models in the planning of nerve-sparing robot-assisted RP have been developed to help achieve more accurate visualization of the NVB [8].

To improve surgical performance and guided by a precision medicine mindset, studies have explored new technologies. For instance, diffusion tensor imaging (DTI), a modality that allows fiber tract reconstruction, has shown promising results in the preoperative scenario [9].

In fact, Sievert et al. [26] described a positive correlation between nerve distribution in functional histologic studies and DTI findings. This MRI biotechnology is based on the sensitivity to diffusion of water protons along the longitudinal direction of myelinated fibers [27, 28]. Although it has long been used in the field of neurosurgery, it is an innovative tool for understanding neural anatomical complexity in prostate cancer.

Intraoperative Considerations

Modified Apical Dissection and Lateral Prostatic Fascial Preservation

In a propensity score-matched analysis [3], the authors modified the conventional approach of RALP with preservation of NVB by dissecting medially to the lateral prostatic fascia and adopting a modified apical dissection. This helps avoid traction and thermal injury to the NVB and preserves the distal levator fibers that interdigitate with the rhabdosphincter of the urethra. This technical modification also involves apical dissection under the puboprostatic ligaments preserving maximum periurethral tissue and avoiding damage to the veins and arteries of the deep venous complex (DVC) and Santorini plexus at the apex. The study resulted in an increased potency rate of 44 and 57% from 21 and 35% at 6 weeks and 3 months, respectively.

Veil of Aphrodite and Superveil Technique

Menon et al. [4, 29] developed the Veil of Aphrodite, also known as the curtain dissection technique, where initially the prostatic capsule is separated from the prostatic fascia starting at the base of SVs using harmonic ACE. The prostatic fascia stays as a supportive overlay on the NVBs, hanging like a curtain from the puboure-thral ligaments. Further, the interfacial plane between the posterior prostatic fascia and the DVF is extended toward the apex at 1 and 5 o'clock for the right side and between 6 and 11 o'clock for the left side. The pedicles are divided and this dissection is continued anteriorly. Preservation of CNs and reduced traction injury are achieved with this technique, ultimately allowing 70% of patients to be able to have intercourse post-RALP with SHIM>21 and who underwent bilateral NS.

Further, with evidence of 25% of nerves present anteriorly, the author modified his technique with an idea to preserve the pubovesical ligaments and DVC. This modification involves extending the interfacial dissection between 11 and 1 o'clock positions. Ninety-four percent of men with the superveil were able to have erections strong enough to have intercourse. Both veil and superveil techniques both had comparable SHIM scores; however, men with superveil had earlier return of potency [5].

Retrograde Versus Antegrade Release of NVBs

In the retrograde release of the NVB, the initial dissection with 0° lens of the anterior peritoneum, using a 30° lens turned downward the anterior bladder neck, is incised without opening the endopelvic fascia followed by the posterior bladder neck. The DVF is incised and posterior dissection is done. In this technique, release of the NVB is at the bladder neck, and an avascular plane is created under the DVC. Turning the 30° lens up, further lateral dissection is carried out considering the anatomical boundaries of the NVB. NS was performed using the prostate artery. The prostatic apex is dissected underneath the DVC, with an aim of preserving maximum urethral stump, followed by posterior reconstruction of the rhabdosphincter, endopelvic fascia, and peri-prostatic collar reconstruction. This modification helped the authors spare the anterior prostatic nerves and vessels by retrograde release of the NVB with preservation of the DVC.

Carvalho et al. [6] in this study demonstrate good functional outcomes, especially in terms of EF with 53% of patients accomplishing potency after 1 month and 69.9% and 86.7% after 3 and 12 months, respectively. Further, Patel et al. [30] described athermal retrograde release of the NVB with minimal traction where NS is performed using the prostate artery, toward the prostatic base. The prostatic pedicles are clipped at last, resulting in a traction-free natural release of the NVB. Their study showed that 87.7% men with SHIM >21 and 73% men with SHIM 17–21 were potent at 3 months post-surgery.

In the antegrade approach of NS, after gentle traction on the vas and SV, countertraction is applied on the prostate. This exposes a triangular space bounded by the prostatic fascia, lateral prostatic fascia, and DVF, which serves as a landmark for inter-/intrafascial dissection [31].

Comparing both these aforementioned techniques, a questionnaire-based assessment of the antegrade approach of NS showed more men to be potent as compared to the retrograde approach, but these results were from open/laparoscopic RP. On the contrary, Ko et al. [32] in his study of men undergoing RALP demonstrate significantly higher potency rates at 3, 6, and 9 months with the retrograde approach of NS.

NS Dissection: Unilateral Versus Bilateral (b/l), Athermal Versus Monopolar Versus Bipolar, and Pedicle Control (Clips or Clipless Techniques)

Several studies in the last few decades have taken into consideration the dissection technique, energy, and instruments used for dissection that affect potency outcomes on a short- and long-term basis. Ahlering et al. [33] found a delayed potency return after the use of bipolar and monopolar electrocautery in the NVB dissection or vascular pedicle transection.

A systematic review and meta-analysis concluded that b/l NS, intrafascial dissection/maximum NVB, and peri-prostatic tissue preservation via grade 1 NS dissection helped achieve the best potency rate and oncological outcomes [34]. This meta-analysis supports a cautery-free technique or use of pinpoint low-energy cauterization for dissection of the NVB and peri-prostatic planes. Moreover, many of the above study results involve clipless technique and have shown early return of potency. These studies suggest that the potential damage caused by the use of mono-/bipolar dissection can be minimized by longer follow-up, particularly in young patients. These results are further supported by the study, showing good potency rates at 24-month follow-up [35] (Video 5.1).

Use of Energy and Avoiding Countertraction on NVB During RALP

The nerves in the NVB are sensitive to thermal injury caused by the thermal dissection, and damage to these nerves causes loss of EF post-RALP. Hence, cautery-free techniques focusing on achieving hemostasis and minimal injury to the NVB are used. These include vascular clips, suture ligation, bulldog clamps, and other sealing substances. Falgin et al. [36] compared the potency outcomes post-RALP using three different techniques of dissecting the NVB: series 1, utilized selective bipolar cautery for NS; series 2, used an athermal "clip and peel" posterior dissection technique; and series 3, used an athermal combined anterior and posterior dissection technique with clips and sharp dissection alone. The study demonstrates that series 3 has superior potency rate at 3 months post-RALP and minimal PSMs.

Moreover, irreversible tissue injuries are related to the use of temperatures >58 °C. Mandhani et al. [37] performed intraoperative thermal mapping around the

NVB wherein they recorded the temperature changes around the NVB during dissection. They found that the temperature changes in cases using an athermal dissection, compared to those undergoing a non-NS surgery. In the former group, monopolar dissection was associated with an average increase in temperature up to 43.68 °C (36.4–47.38 °C), whereas with the bipolar dissection, the average temperature registered was 38.88 °C (36.88–42.68 °C). Interestingly, during the non-NS surgery, temperatures were higher with the bipolar energy (47.2–109.88 °C, mean 60.918 °C), exceeding the safety values for tissue preservation. Furthermore, the time to reach a nadir temperature was also longer with the bipolar energy (6.4 vs. 3.4 s). This study suggested that bipolar cautery is not safer than monopolar cautery, with a potential impact on tissues within 1 cm from the place where the energy is applied. Consequently, it should be avoided close to the NVB.

Another study by Mattie et al. [38] performed a tension-free RALP with interfacial dissection of the NVB, where good potency outcomes were noted. 64.5% of the patients were found to have total SHIM scores of 17, and 17.2% of them scored 26. In their technique, after mobilization of fat from the prostate and exposing the endopelvic fascia, they separated the bladder neck from the prostatic base. After isolation of the right pedicle, dissection begins at the prostatic base, endopelvic fascia, and peri-prostatic fascia are opened at 2 o'clock. Using blunt dissection, the prostate is separated along its lateral border until the NVB is reached. This dissection continues to the apex and the right SV is mobilized. Similar dissection is performed on the left side until the urethra is reached. After this posterior and lateral dissection, the prostate can be viewed dorsally, Santorini's plexus and the urethra are transected, and hemostasis of Santorini's plexus is achieved using a vertical stitch. A vesicourethral anastomosis is done.

A more recent study by Kowalczyk et al. [39] involved application of assistant suction tip on the right NVB, and robotic Maryland dissector applied countertraction to the left NVB to facilitate prostatic dissection away from the NVB instead of the NVB dissection away from the prostate. Countertraction on NVB leads to neuropraxia and delayed recovery of sexual function, and this study showed early return of sexual function and potency at 5 months with avoidance of countertraction.

Dehydrated Human Amnion/Chorion Membrane (dHAM) Wrap Around the NVB for Neuroprotection and Early Nerve Regeneration

Human amniotic membrane is a composite non-immunogenic tissue consisting of cytokines, growth factors, and neurotrophic factors that play a pivotal role in regressing the inflammatory process, regeneration of the neuronal tissue through its stem cell-like properties [40, 41], preventing fibrosis of the traumatic tissues, and promoting healing following traumatic and thermal/athermal injury [42, 43].

dHAM is derived from the consensually donated human placenta of screened and tested women obtained during a C-section according to the American Association of Tissue Banks standards and is considered a tissue product under

Section 361 of the Public Health Service Act. This biologically active amniotic tissue membrane is stored as manipulated, cleaned, dehydrated, and sterilized sheets, wraps, particulate, and membrane configurations for medicinal use. Its safety and use in humans and experimental animals have been well documented in the literature for wound healing and nerve regeneration [44].

Pioneering the usage of dHAM in the field of Urology, Razdan et al. used a dHAM allograft nerve sheet as a wrap (AmnioFix™ of size 6 cm × 6 cm; BU-5660, MiMedx Group Inc., Marietta, GA, USA) around the NVB (31st World Congress of Endourology, Taipei, 2014). The authors demonstrated promising results of early return of continence in a high-volume, single-institution, single-surgeon non-randomized study [45].

Two study groups, matched with age, body mass index, AUA score, prostate-specific antigen, clinical stage, baseline sexual function, Charlson comorbidity index, and NS status, were selected as intervention (with the use of dHAM) and control (without the use of dHAM). All the study participants in the intervention and control group underwent full athermal intrafascial clipless complete b/l NS RALP, with or without dHAM allograft wrapped around the NVBs, respectively. This was followed by the Van Velthoven anastomosis and preserving maximum urethral length. The primary endpoint of time taken to return to predefined degrees of potency was significantly less in the intervention group, and the secondary objective of the quantal change in potency (at 3 monthly intervals until 1 year post-RALP), subjectively manifested as the difference in sexual health inventory for men (SHIM) questionnaire score (ΔSHIM score), was significantly lower too in the intervention group as compared to the control group. More men in the intervention group were achieving potency every quarter than in the control group. The results were monitored telephonically every month and with a clinical visit follow-up every 3 months, with some international patients being closely followed up telephonically. Most of the patients achieved potency at 3 months' time interval following surgery, with potency rates higher at 3-, 6-, 9- and 12-month follow-up in the intervention group.

The results of this study are further supported by many subsequent studies [46, 47], which demonstrate similar results of significantly lower mean time of potency recovery in the group with graft wrapped around the NVB as compared to the control group, in all grades of NS performed.

The Menon Precision Prostatectomy (MPP)

This novel surgical technique was recently proposed by Sood et al. [48]. It involves preservation of the SV and a 5–10 mm rim of prostatic capsule contralateral to the dominant lesion. This technique has reported promising preliminary outcomes in eight patients, who achieved potency within 12 months of surgery and continence within 4 months. A prospective randomized clinical trial currently being conducted will provide more data concerning oncological safety and functional results [48].

NVB Alignment Around SV and SV Preservation

Ganzer et al. [49] in adult male cadavers found the number of capsular nerves increased significantly from the base over the middle to the apex, with a total of 983, 1825, and 2057 nerves, respectively ($p < 0.001$). Majority of nerves run at the posterolateral surface of SVs. Planimetry studies have demonstrated 75% of nerves from the SVs do not reach the striated urethral sphincter and innervate structures other than the CC.

Muroka et al. [50] through immunohistochemistry staining of male cadavers found that the nerves in all the proposed groups of nerve bundles around the SV are sympathetic in nature: anterosuperior between the bladder and SV and middle and superior between the SV and rectum.

Several observational studies have found that SV preservation helps avoid NVB injury and gives better functional outcomes [51, 52]. However, a small randomized controlled trial contradicts this finding, showing no difference in functional recovery in both the comparison groups [53].

Locoregional Hypothermia of the Pelvis

Using an endorectal cooling balloon to generate hypothermia reduces inflammatory injury. One study utilized endorectal cooling balloon and cold irrigation to generate hypothermia. This began before incision until the patient was ready to return to the recovery room, with intermittent pauses during anastomosis or rectal dissection due to space limitation. This novel technique significantly provided potency rate of 83 vs. 66% in the control group. However, a prospective controlled trial needs to confirm the reliability of this advancement [54].

Avoiding Ischemic Stress to Penis (Continuous Oxygen Monitoring)

Several additional advancements have been tried during NS with a goal of better handling and decreasing the stress on the NVB. Tewari et al. [55] used intraoperative continuous oxygen monitoring to demonstrate ischemic stress to the penis, especially during NS, endopelvic fascial opening, retraction of the prostate as well as Foley catheter, and SV traction. This led to adjustments in tissue handling during surgery and achieving better functional outcomes.

Following Visual Cues Intraoperatively

Schatloff et al. [20] followed visual cues intraoperatively to identify the prostate artery that helped achieve more consistent NS during RALP. This grading system considers unilateral NS, lateral traction on NVB, peri-prostatic adhesions, athermal hemostasis, trauma to NVB, and bleeding >100 ml to give a score. This has been further found to be the single most important predictor in achieving potency at 1 year [56].

Hydro-dissection of NVBs

Pedraza et al. [57] developed an innovative NS technique known as saline-assisted fascial engorgement (SAFE) guided by micro-ultrasound (MUS). In this technique, after the early release of the NVB, a plane between the DVF and prostatic capsule is identified, and a 20 ml of normal saline solution is infused from the apex to the base using the micro-ultrasound. Men who underwent the SAFE technique had higher SHIM score compared to the control group at 6-week and 3-month follow-up.

Guru et al. [58] also demonstrated similar technique of hydro-dissecting the NVB for better NVB preservation. This study used 1:10,000 epinephrine solution diluted in 0.9% normal saline into the lateral prostatic pedicle with an injection cannula needle (Wolf). The intraoperative parameters were favorable; however, EF outcomes were awaiting long-term follow-up.

Role of Laser in NS

Studies have demonstrated the use of lasers wherein CO_2 is used to create a plane between the prostatic capsule and NVB to facilitate a meticulous NS [59]. The laser used was the OmniGuide® BeamPathTM URO-LG CO2 laser fiber by Cheetham et al. [59]. CO_2 lasers increase temperature up to a maximum of 40 °C, with a minimal thermal energy up to the 0.5 mm vicinity of the dissection tissue. This study demonstrated promising continence results at 3-month post-RALP. Potency was not evaluated.

Another study evaluated CN function using KTP laser dissection and compared the outcomes with ultrasonic shears and cold scissor dissection [60]. The authors assessed median peak intracavernous pressure as a percent of mean arterial pressure, and results were in favor of the KTP and were comparable to athermal technique of dissection. However, these findings were in a laparoscopic RP setting, and the results will need to be validated in the RALP setting.

Devices for Identifying the Cavernous Nerves Intraoperatively: Electrical Nerve Stimulation and the Role of Near-Infrared Fluorescence (NIRF) and Indocyanine Green (ICG)

Over the past few decades, many devices have been applied intraoperatively for CN visualization. These include electrical nerve stimulation devices, fluorescence imaging, and TRUS. Electrical nerve stimulation induces erectile response in the penis, and the change in the circumference of the penis (tumescence) is measured as a sign of correct probe placement on the CN by the surgeon. Though the Cavermap devices have been found to be effective in nerve identification and stimulation, the results for positive impact on potency rates or time to potency return remains controversial and still needs further investigations [61–65].

Another electrical nerve stimulation device is the fixed bipolar electrode. Intracavernous response or intraurethral pressure was measured to identify CNs. Results of this study were significantly associated with EF [46].

Fluorescein and indocyanine green are FDA-approved dyes frequently used in studies either by local injection into the cavernous nerve via the penis or systemic route via intravenous injection. Kumar et al. [66] used ICG to identify the landmark prostatic artery by IV injection of the dye. The dye emits green florescence under an infrared laser that is picked up by the endoscope signal detector and relayed to the robotic console for visualization by the surgeon. The landmark artery is visualized as a green fluorescent vessel on the lateral prostate. The use of these dyes has been well documented as a successful tool to identify peri-prostatic vessels and cancerous areas around the prostate that indirectly help achieve better NS and oncological outcomes [67–69]. However, more research is needed in this area to identify the CN and NVB directly, and studies need to evaluate EF using this modality.

Intraoperative Monitoring of CN Response

Song et al. [70] completed a successful feasibility study on intraoperative monitoring of CN response via spontaneously evoked median nerve stimulation and NVB-triggered corpora cavernosa electromyography. The authors showed a positive correlation with the baseline EF and also predicted its recovery after surgery. However, feasibility of these findings for incorporation into daily practice needs further investigation.

Conclusion

Numerous intraoperative techniques have been described in the literature to optimize early return of EF during RALP. These techniques stem from proper understanding of cavernous and NVB anatomy and the fascial layers of the prostate and also incorporate preoperative imaging to better gauge the relevant neural anatomy.

Take-Home Message

This chapter covers the wide breadth of intraoperative techniques that can be utilized to optimize postoperative erectile function after RALP. These techniques encompass athermal dissection of cavernous nerves, hydrodissection of fascial layers, and prospective identification with nerve stimulation and lasers. As described at the start of this chapter, effective adoption of these techniques stems from careful study of the prostatic and pelvic anatomy. The surgeon has a large arsenal of techniques to choose from based on the available literature to prevent nerve damage and postop ED. While availability of certain technologies may be limited in practice, prospective identification of nerve bundles and limiting thermal nerve injury and neuropraxia serves as the mainstay of all described innovations.

References

1. Walsh PC, Donker PJ. Impotence following radical prostatectomy: insight into etiology and prevention. J Urol. 1982;128(3):492–7.
2. Nyangoh Timoh K, Moszkowicz D, Creze M, Zaitouna M, Felber M, Lebacle C, et al. The male external urethral sphincter is autonomically innervated. Clin Anat. 2021;34(2):263–71.
3. Covas Moschovas M, Bhat S, Onol FF, Rogers T, Roof S, Mazzone E, et al. Modified apical dissection and lateral prostatic fascia preservation improves early postoperative functional recovery in robotic-assisted laparoscopic radical prostatectomy: results from a propensity score-matched analysis. Eur Urol. 2020;78(6):875–84.
4. Kaul S, Savera A, Badani K, Fumo M, Bhandari A, Menon M. Functional outcomes and oncological efficacy of Vattikuti Institute prostatectomy with Veil of Aphrodite nerve-sparing: an analysis of 154 consecutive patients. BJU Int. 2006;97(3):467–72.
5. Menon M, Shrivastava A, Bhandari M, Satyanarayana R, Siva S, Agarwal PK. Vattikuti Institute prostatectomy: technical modifications in 2009. Eur Urol. 2009;56(1):89–96.
6. Montorsi F, Gandaglia G, Würnschimmel C, Graefen M, Briganti A, Huland H. Re: Paolo Afonso de Carvalho, João A.B.A. Barbosa, Giuliano B. Guglielmetti, et al. Retrograde release of the neurovascular bundle with preservation of dorsal venous complex during robot-assisted radical prostatectomy: optimizing functional outcomes. Eur Urol. 2020;77:628–35: incredible results for robot-assisted nerve-sparing radical prostatectomy in prostate cancer patients. Eur Urol. 2021;79(2):e44–e6.
7. KleinJan GH, Sikorska K, Korne CM, Brouwer OR, Buckle T, Tillier C, et al. A prediction model relating the extent of intraoperative fascia preservation to erectile dysfunction after nerve-sparing robot-assisted radical prostatectomy. J Robot Surg. 2019;13(3):455–62.
8. Veerman H, Boellaard TN, van der Eijk JA, Sluijter JH, Roeleveld TA, van der Sluis TM, et al. Development and clinical applicability of MRI-based 3D prostate models in the planning of nerve-sparing robot-assisted radical prostatectomy. J Robot Surg. 2022;2:509–17.
9. Panebianco V, Barchetti F, Sciarra A, Marcantonio A, Zini C, Salciccia S, et al. In vivo 3D neuroanatomical evaluation of periprostatic nerve plexus with 3T-MR diffusion tensor imaging. Eur J Radiol. 2013;82(10):1677–82.
10. Mulhall JP, Klein EA, Slawin K, Henning AK, Scardino PT. A randomized, double-blind, placebo-controlled trial to assess the utility of tacrolimus (FK506) for the prevention of erectile dysfunction following bilateral nerve-sparing radical prostatectomy. J Sex Med. 2018;15(9):1293–9.
11. Yoshimura N, Kato R, Chancellor MB, Nelson JB, Glorioso JC. Gene therapy as future treatment of erectile dysfunction. Expert Opin Biol Ther. 2010;10(9):1305–14.
12. Tewari A, Takenaka A, Mtui E, Horninger W, Peschel R, Bartsch G, et al. The proximal neurovascular plate and the tri-zonal neural architecture around the prostate gland: importance in the athermal robotic technique of nerve-sparing prostatectomy. BJU Int. 2006;98(2):314–23.
13. Takenaka A, Murakami G, Soga H, Han SH, Arai Y, Fujisawa M. Anatomical analysis of the neurovascular bundle supplying penile cavernous tissue to ensure a reliable nerve graft after radical prostatectomy. J Urol. 2004;172(3):1032–5.
14. Lunacek A, Schwentner C, Fritsch H, Bartsch G, Strasser H. Anatomical radical retropubic prostatectomy: 'curtain dissection' of the neurovascular bundle. BJU Int. 2005;95(9):1226–31.
15. Kaiho Y, Nakagawa H, Saito H, Ito A, Ishidoya S, Saito S, et al. Nerves at the ventral prostatic capsule contribute to erectile function: initial electrophysiological assessment in humans. Eur Urol. 2009;55(1):148–54.

16. Han M, Trock BJ, Partin AW, Humphreys EB, Bivalacqua TJ, Guzzo TJ, et al. The impact of preoperative erectile dysfunction on survival after radical prostatectomy. BJU Int. 2010;106(11):1612–7.
17. Takenaka A, Kawada M, Murakami G, Hisasue S, Tsukamoto T, Fujisawa M. Interindividual variation in distribution of extramural ganglion cells in the male pelvis: a semi-quantitative and immunohistochemical study concerning nerve-sparing pelvic surgery. Eur Urol. 2005;48(1):46–52; discussion.
18. Walz J, Epstein JI, Ganzer R, Graefen M, Guazzoni G, Kaouk J, et al. A critical analysis of the current knowledge of surgical anatomy of the prostate related to optimisation of cancer control and preservation of continence and erection in candidates for radical prostatectomy: an update. Eur Urol. 2016;70(2):301–11.
19. Wagaskar VG, Mittal A, Sobotka S, Ratnani P, Lantz A, Falagario UG, et al. Hood technique for robotic radical prostatectomy-preserving periurethral anatomical structures in the space of Retzius and sparing the pouch of Douglas, enabling early return of continence without compromising surgical margin rates. Eur Urol. 2021;80(2):213–21.
20. Schatloff O, Chauhan S, Sivaraman A, Kameh D, Palmer KJ, Patel VR. Anatomic grading of nerve sparing during robot-assisted radical prostatectomy. Eur Urol. 2012;61(4):796–802.
21. Tewari AK, Srivastava A, Huang MW, Robinson BD, Shevchuk MM, Durand M, et al. Anatomical grades of nerve sparing: a risk-stratified approach to neural-hammock sparing during robot-assisted radical prostatectomy (RARP). BJU Int. 2011;108(6 Pt 2):984–92.
22. Tewari A, Grover S, Sooriakumaran P, Srivastava A, Rao S, Gupta A, et al. Nerve sparing can preserve orgasmic function in most men after robotic-assisted laparoscopic radical prostatectomy. BJU Int. 2012;109(4):596–602.
23. Montorsi F, Wilson TG, Rosen RC, Ahlering TE, Artibani W, Carroll PR, et al. Best practices in robot-assisted radical prostatectomy: recommendations of the Pasadena Consensus Panel. Eur Urol. 2012;62(3):368–81.
24. Stolzenburg JU, Kallidonis P, Do M, Dietel A, Häfner T, Rabenalt R, et al. A comparison of outcomes for interfascial and intrafascial nerve-sparing radical prostatectomy. Urology. 2010;76(3):743–8.
25. Kozikowski M, Malewski W, Michalak W, Dobruch J. Clinical utility of MRI in the decision-making process before radical prostatectomy: systematic review and meta-analysis. PLoS One. 2019;14(1):e0210194.
26. Sievert KD, Hennenlotter J, Dillenburg T, Toomey P, Wöllner J, Zweers P, et al. Extended periprostatic nerve distributions on the prostate surface confirmed using diffusion tensor imaging. BJU Int. 2019;123(6):995–1004.
27. Garcia-Monaco R, Garategui L, Kizilevsky N, Peralta O, Rodriguez P, Palacios-Jaraquemada J. Human cadaveric specimen study of the prostatic arterial anatomy: implications for arterial embolization. J Vasc Interv Radiol. 2014;25(2):315–22.
28. Fine SW, Reuter VE. Anatomy of the prostate revisited: implications for prostate biopsy and zonal origins of prostate cancer. Histopathology. 2012;60(1):142–52.
29. Menon M, Shrivastava A, Kaul S, Badani KK, Fumo M, Bhandari M, et al. Vattikuti Institute prostatectomy: contemporary technique and analysis of results. Eur Urol 2007;51(3):648–57; discussion 57–8.
30. Coughlin G, Dangle PP, Palmer KJ, Samevedi S, Patel VR. Athermal early retrograde release of the neurovascular bundle during nerve-sparing robotic-assisted laparoscopic radical prostatectomy. J Robot Surg. 2009;3(1):13–7.
31. Carini M, Masieri L, Minervini A, Lapini A, Serni S. Oncological and functional results of antegrade radical retropubic prostatectomy for the treatment of clinically localised prostate cancer. Eur Urol. 2008;53(3):554–61.
32. Ko YH, Coelho RF, Sivaraman A, Schatloff O, Chauhan S, Abdul-Muhsin HM, et al. Retrograde versus antegrade nerve sparing during robot-assisted radical prostatectomy: which is better for achieving early functional recovery? Eur Urol. 2013;63(1):169–77.
33. Ahlering TE, Eichel L, Skarecky D. Evaluation of long-term thermal injury using cautery during nerve sparing robotic prostatectomy. Urology. 2008;72(6):1371–4.

34. Ficarra V, Novara G, Ahlering TE, Costello A, Eastham JA, Graefen M, et al. Systematic review and meta-analysis of studies reporting potency rates after robot-assisted radical prostatectomy. Eur Urol. 2012;62(3):418–30.
35. Novara G, Ficarra V, D'Elia C, Secco S, De Gobbi A, Cavalleri S, et al. Preoperative criteria to select patients for bilateral nerve-sparing robotic-assisted radical prostatectomy. J Sex Med. 2010;7(2 Pt 1):839–45.
36. Da FR. Vinci prostatectomy: athermal nerve sparing and effect of the technique on erectile recovery and negative margins. J Robot Surg. 2007;1(2):139–43.
37. Mandhani A, Dorsey PJ, Ramanathan R, Salamanca JI, Rao S, Leung R, et al. Real time monitoring of temperature changes in neurovascular bundles during robotic radical prostatectomy: thermal map for nerve-sparing radical prostatectomy. J Endourol. 2008;22(10):2313–7.
38. Mattei A, Naspro R, Annino F, Burke D, Guida R, Gaston R. Tension and energy-free robotic-assisted laparoscopic radical prostatectomy with interfascial dissection of the neurovascular bundles. Eur Urol. 2007;52(3):687–94.
39. Kowalczyk KJ, Huang AC, Hevelone ND, Lipsitz SR, Yu HY, Ulmer WD, et al. Stepwise approach for nerve sparing without countertraction during robot-assisted radical prostatectomy: technique and outcomes. Eur Urol. 2011;60(3):536–47.
40. Ricciardelli G, Ceccuzzi R, Raneri M, Scalisi A, Bianchi PE. Management of recurrent corneal ulcers: use of amniotic membrane. Eur J Ophthalmol. 2014;24(5):793–6.
41. Massee M, Chinn K, Lei J, Lim JJ, Young CS, Koob TJ. Dehydrated human amnion/chorion membrane regulates stem cell activity in vitro. J Biomed Mater Res B Appl Biomater. 2016;104(7):1495–503.
42. Fetterolf DE, Snyder RJ. Scientific and clinical support for the use of dehydrated amniotic membrane in wound management. Wounds. 2012;24(10):299–307.
43. Zelen CM, Gould L, Serena TE, Carter MJ, Keller J, Li WW. A prospective, randomised, controlled, multi-centre comparative effectiveness study of healing using dehydrated human amnion/chorion membrane allograft, bioengineered skin substitute or standard of care for treatment of chronic lower extremity diabetic ulcers. Int Wound J. 2015;12(6):724–32.
44. Ogaya-Pinies G, Palayapalam-Ganapathi H, Rogers T, Hernandez-Cardona E, Rocco B, Coelho RF, et al. Can dehydrated human amnion/chorion membrane accelerate the return to potency after a nerve-sparing robotic-assisted radical prostatectomy? Propensity score-matched analysis. J Robot Surg. 2018;12(2):235–43.
45. Razdan S, Bajpai RR, Sanchez MA. A matched and controlled longitudinal cohort study of dehydrated human amniotic membrane allograft sheet used as a wraparound nerve bundles in robotic-assisted laparoscopic radical prostatectomy: a puissant adjunct for enhanced potency outcomes. J Robot Surg. 2019;13(3):475–81.
46. Krol BC, Hemal AK, Peak T, Liu S, Pathak RA. Early return to continence and potency with use of dehydrated human umbilical cord graft at the time of robot-assisted radical prostatectomy: a case study and analysis of relevant literature. IJU Case Rep. 2021;4(3):151–3.
47. Noël J, Mascarenhas A, Patel E, Reddy S, Sandri M, Bhat S, et al. Nerve spare robot assisted laparoscopic prostatectomy with amniotic membranes: medium term outcomes. J Robot Surg. 2022;16(5):1219–24.
48. Sood A, Abdollah F, Jeong W, Menon M. The precision prostatectomy: "waiting for Godot". Eur Urol Focus. 2020;6(2):227–30.
49. Ganzer R, Blana A, Gaumann A, Stolzenburg JU, Rabenalt R, Bach T, et al. Topographical anatomy of periprostatic and capsular nerves: quantification and computerised planimetry. Eur Urol. 2008;54(2):353–60.
50. Muraoka K, Morizane S, Hieda K, Honda M, Sejima T, Murakami G, et al. Site-dependent differences in the composite fibers of male pelvic plexus branches: an immunohistochemical analysis of donated elderly cadavers. BMC Urol. 2018;18(1):47.
51. John H, Hauri D. Seminal vesicle-sparing radical prostatectomy: a novel concept to restore early urinary continence. Urology. 2000;55(6):820–4.

52. Albers P, Schäfers S, Löhmer H, de Geeter P. Seminal vesicle-sparing perineal radical prostatectomy improves early functional results in patients with low-risk prostate cancer. BJU Int. 2007;100(5):1050–4.
53. Gilbert SM, Dunn RL, Miller DC, Montgomery JS, Skolarus TA, Weizer AZ, et al. Functional outcomes following nerve sparing prostatectomy augmented with seminal vesicle sparing compared to standard nerve sparing prostatectomy: results from a randomized controlled trial. J Urol. 2017;198(3):600–7.
54. Finley DS, Chang A, Morales B, Osann K, Skarecky D, Ahlering T. Impact of regional hypothermia on urinary continence and potency after robot-assisted radical prostatectomy. J Endourol. 2010;24(7):1111–6.
55. Tewari A, Srivastava A, Sooriakumaran P, Grover S, Dorsey P, Leung R. Technique of traction-free nerve-sparing robotic prostatectomy: delicate tissue handling by real-time penile oxygen monitoring. Int J Impot Res. 2012;24(1):11–9.
56. Bajpai RR, Razdan S, Sanchez MA. A novel intraoperative physician-assigned grading score to predict postoperative return of potency at 1 year after robotic-assisted laparoscopic prostatectomy. Indian J Urol. 2019;35(1):61–6.
57. Pedraza AM, Parekh S, Joshi H, Grauer R, Wagaskar V, Zuluaga L, et al. Side-specific, microultrasound-based nomogram for the prediction of extracapsular extension in prostate cancer. Eur Urol Open Sci. 2023;48:72–81.
58. Guru KA, Perlmutter AE, Butt ZM, Peabody JO. Hydrodissection for preservation of neurovascular bundle during robot-assisted radical prostatectomy. Can J Urol. 2008;15(2):4000–3.
59. Cheetham PJ, Truesdale MD, Lee DJ, Landman JM, Badani KK. Use of a flexible carbon dioxide laser fiber for precise dissection of the neurovascular bundle during robot-assisted laparoscopic prostatectomy. J Endourol. 2010;24(7):1091–6.
60. Gianduzzo TR, Colombo JR, Haber GP, Magi-Galluzzi C, Dall'Oglio MF, Ulchaker J, et al. KTP laser nerve sparing radical prostatectomy: comparison of ultrasonic and cold scissor dissection on cavernous nerve function. J Urol. 2009;181(6):2760–6.
61. Kaiho Y, Ito J, Iwamura H, Anan G, Kuromoto A, Kudo T, et al. Nerves in the areas posterior to the prostate base contribute to erectile function: an intraoperative electrical stimulation assessment. Urology. 2019;132:156–60.
62. Takenaka A, Tewari A, Hara R, Leung RA, Kurokawa K, Murakami G, et al. Pelvic autonomic nerve mapping around the prostate by intraoperative electrical stimulation with simultaneous measurement of intracavernous and intraurethral pressure. J Urol. 2007;177(1):225–9; discussion 9.
63. Kurokawa K, Suzuki T, Suzuki K, Ito K, Shimizu N, Fukabori Y, et al. A simple and reliable monitoring system to confirm the preservation of the cavernous nerves. Int J Urol. 2001;8(5):231–6.
64. Walsh PC, Marschke P, Catalona WJ, Lepor H, Martin S, Myers RP, et al. Efficacy of first-generation Cavermap to verify location and function of cavernous nerves during radical prostatectomy: a multi-institutional evaluation by experienced surgeons. Urology. 2001;57(3):491–4.
65. Klotz L, Heaton J, Jewett M, Chin J, Fleshner N, Goldenberg L, et al. A randomized phase 3 study of intraoperative cavernous nerve stimulation with penile tumescence monitoring to improve nerve sparing during radical prostatectomy. J Urol. 2000;164(5):1573–8.
66. Bates AS, Patel VR. Applications of indocyanine green in robotic urology. J Robot Surg. 2016;10(4):357–9.
67. Fukuhara H, Inoue K, Satake H, Tamura K, Karashima T, Yamasaki I, et al. Photodynamic diagnosis of positive margin during radical prostatectomy: preliminary experience with 5-aminolevulinic acid. Int J Urol. 2011;18(8):585–91.
68. Inoue K, Ashida S, Fukuhara H, Iiyama T, Miyamura M, Kurabayashi A, et al. Application of 5-aminolevulinic acid-mediated photodynamic diagnosis to robot-assisted laparoscopic radical prostatectomy. Urology. 2013;82(5):1175–8.

69. Manny TB, Patel M, Hemal AK. Fluorescence-enhanced robotic radical prostatectomy using real-time lymphangiography and tissue marking with percutaneous injection of unconjugated indocyanine green: the initial clinical experience in 50 patients. Eur Urol. 2014;65(6):1162–8.
70. Song WH, Park JH, Tae BS, Kim SM, Hur M, Seo JH, et al. Establishment of novel intraoperative monitoring and mapping method for the cavernous nerve during robot-assisted radical prostatectomy: results of the phase I/II, first-in-human, feasibility study. Eur Urol. 2020;78(2):221–8.

Technical Innovations and New Therapies to Optimize Functional Outcomes After Radiation Therapy

6

Marisa Kollmeier and Benjamin Silver

Introduction

Radiation therapy (RT), either alone or in combination with other modalities, is routinely utilized in the management of clinically localized, locally advanced, and recurrent prostate cancers with excellent cancer control [1]. Depending on various patient-related and clinicopathologic factors, curative-intent radiation therapy can be broadly defined as external beam radiation therapy (EBRT) or brachytherapy (BT), and each can be used alone or combined for optimal targeting and dose delivery. While these treatments are highly effective for prostate cancer, care must be taken to appropriately select patients and tailor treatment to patient- and disease-specific needs in order to minimize treatment-related sequelae while concurrently optimizing outcome. For the purpose of this discussion, we will focus on techniques to minimize treatment-related impact on urinary and sexual quality of life.

General Effects of Radiation on Tissue

Radiation therapy causes a complex cascade of effects in tissue [2, 3]. The primary mechanism of radiation effects on tumor includes indirect and direct damage to DNA leading to cancer cell death in target tissues. Indirect damage is caused by the formation of reactive oxygen species leading to oxidative double- and single-strand breaks [4, 5]. DNA damage results in altered gene expression and recruitment of

M. Kollmeier (✉)
Department of Radiation Oncology, Memorial Sloan Kettering Cancer Center, New York, NY, USA
e-mail: KollmeiM@mskcc.org

B. Silver
Rochester Regional Health, Rochester, NY, USA

S. Razdan, S. Razdan (eds.), *Urinary Continence and Sexual Function After Robotic Prostatectomy, Radiation, and Novel Therapies*,
https://doi.org/10.1007/978-3-031-64245-6_6

pro-inflammatory cytokines and chemokines such as TNF-α, TGF-β, IL-1, and IL-6 [2, 3, 6]. The resultant acute clinical effects of this inflammatory recruitment are manifested as tissue-specific and dose-dependent inflammation.

As cells are most susceptible to radiation-related cell death during cell division (late G2 and M phase), tissues with rapid cell turnover are more susceptible to acute effects compared to those with slow cell turnover [6]. Examples of tissues with rapid cell turnover include the epidermis of the skin, GI tract epithelium, and hematopoietic cells. Although ionizing radiation damage in these tissues will quickly lead to inflammation, cell hypoplasia, and loss of epithelial function, tissue regeneration will typically occur due to repopulating progenitor stem cells [6].

The inflammatory cascade incited by ionizing radiation ultimately may result in late effects such as fibrosis and angiogenesis due to fibroblast production and conversion to myofibroblasts which produce collagen, fibronectin, and proteoglycans. Fibrosis and telangiectasia formation are the most common manifestations in tissues such as the skin, soft tissue, and epithelium. These effects can vary in severity based on dose, volume, technique, and patient-specific susceptibility [2, 3]. Additionally, ischemia due to epithelial cell damage and fibrosis can cause dose-dependent late effects including poor wound healing. In general, larger fraction size (i.e., dose per radiation treatment delivered) is the dominant factor predicting late effects. Patient-related factors predicting late sequelae include age, comorbid conditions (e.g., diabetes mellitus, connective tissue disorders, and vascular diseases), and concurrent therapies.

Urinary Functional Outcomes

Urinary dysfunction following radiation therapy can be multifactorial, and it is fundamental to toxicity mitigation to have a complete understanding of baseline urinary function and predisposing risk factors for the individual patient. Patient-reported outcome assessment should be performed using validated tools such as the International Prostate Symptom Score (IPSS) or EPIC Urinary Domain. Pretreatment anatomic variations including benign prostatic hypertrophy changes, the presence or absence of a protuberant median lobe, dense prostatic calcifications, and/or pretreatment tissue defects (e.g., TURP) are important to appreciate and may impact the selected RT technique. Pretreatment urodynamic testing for patients with moderate to severe pretreatment lower urinary tract symptoms is helpful to optimize pre- and posttreatment symptom management. For post-prostatectomy patients, ideally resolution/plateau of urinary incontinence would precede initiation of adjuvant or salvage radiation approaches. In fact, randomized trials examining the role of adjuvant radiation post-prostatectomy allowed a 3–6-month recovery window [7–9]. Comorbidities that may contribute to toxicity risk should be noted. For example, Kalakota et al. reported a greater incidence of late GU toxicity (relative risk 1.36 for grade $\geq$ 2 and relative risk 2.74 for grade $\geq$ 3) in patients with preexisting diabetes mellitus treated with curative-intent EBRT [10]. In a large meta-analysis, higher grade 2 and 3 toxicities were noted in patients with collagen vascular disease

(CVD) in patients receiving radiation, depending on the CVD type, treatment location, and dose [11].

External Beam Radiation Therapy

Urinary morbidities following EBRT can be subdivided into acute (<90 days) and late (≥90 days) toxicities. Acute urinary toxicities (typically irritative/obstructive symptoms) are common (30–50%) and typically begin about 2–3 weeks from initiation of EBRT with peak symptoms at/following treatment completion. Management typically includes the use of alpha blockers, anticholinergics, anti-inflammatories, and/or urinary anesthetics as indicated [12]. Symptom resolution occurs over the weeks following treatment, and most patients return to baseline within 3–6 months following treatment. The incidence of late grade 3 or higher urinary sequelae with radiation therapy ranges from 2% to 5% in the definitive setting [13–15] and 5% to 8% in the postoperative setting [8, 9, 16]. Zaorsky et al. conducted a review of outcomes and toxicities among radiation therapy treatment options for prostate cancer, including 16 studies implementing EBRT [17]. In this review, <1% of patients undergoing definitive EBRT experienced early or late grade 3–4 urinary incontinence, whereas in the post-RP setting, >5% experienced early grade 3–4 incontinence and 1–5% experienced late grade 3–4 incontinence. Further, 1–5% of patients in this review undergoing definitive EBRT experienced early grade 3–4 irritative/obstructive urinary symptoms with <1% experiencing these as late effects. In the post-RP setting, >5% of patients reported early irritative/obstructive urinary toxicity, and <1% of patients reported these as late effects [17]. Generally, late urethral strictures are a concern following EBRT; however, the reported incidence in the SPCG-7/SFUO-3 phase III trial that included 875 men from 47 Scandinavian centers with locally advanced prostate cancer receiving androgen deprivation therapy (ADT) with or without EBRT and found that men receiving ADT with EBRT had a 2% rate of urinary strictures as compared to 0% in the men receiving ADT alone [18].

Optimizing treatment-related toxicity begins with the planning process. When planning an external beam radiation approach, a simulation is performed in the treatment planning position, often with a thermoplastic immobilization device. Following patient positioning, a CT and/or MRI is performed, and treatment planning software is used to delineate target tissues and organs at risk (OARs). MRI has the advantage of better soft tissue delineation and improved visualization of the apex of the prostate to avoid encompassing the external urinary sphincter and pelvic floor musculature (Fig. 6.1). Several techniques may be employed depending on the clinical scenario to displace a normal tissue. Patients may be instructed to fill their bladder prior to treatment to displace portions of the bladder and bowel away from the region of the prostate. Rectal preparations may be employed to empty the rectum to reduce rectal dose. Prior to simulation, a hydrogel rectal spacer can be injected in the retroprostatic space to further displace the rectal wall (Fig. 6.2). In a phase III trial, the use of a rectal spacer during RT reduced 3-year incidence of grade ≥1 and ≥2 rectal toxicity from 9% to 2% and from 6% to 0%, respectively

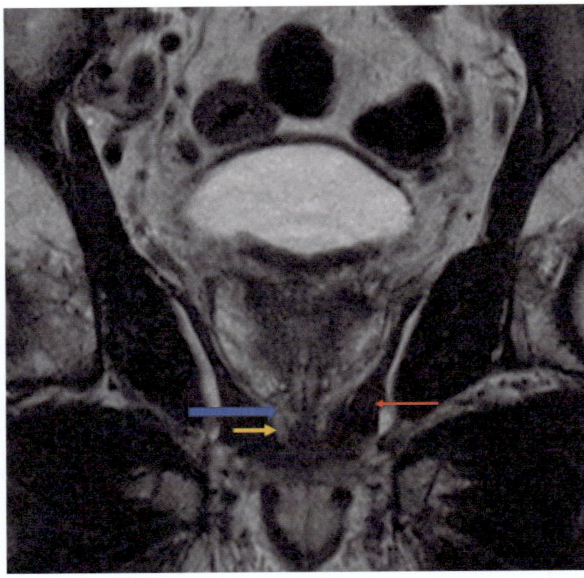

Fig. 6.1 Coronal T2 image of the prostate and adjacent tissue. The prostate apex (blue arrow) is noted below which lies the external urinary sphincter (orange arrow). Red arrow indicates the levator ani muscle

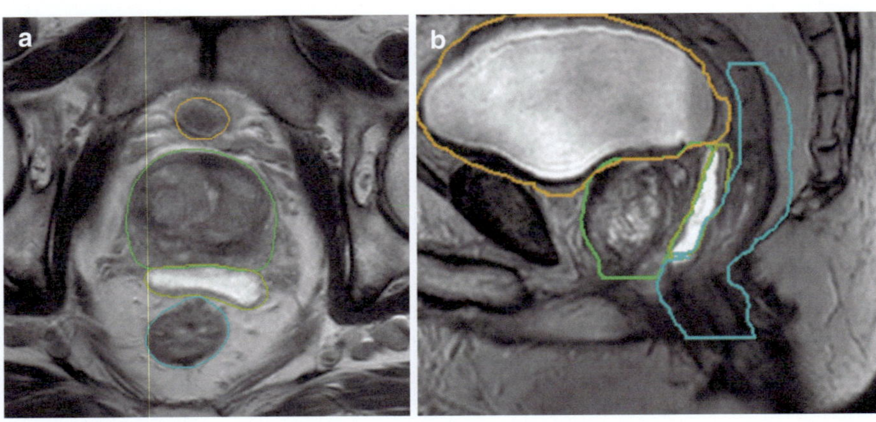

Fig. 6.2 (**a**, **b**) Treatment planning axial (**a**) and sagittal (**b**) T2 MRI with contours draw delineating the prostate (green), rectal spacer (gold), bladder (orange), and rectum (cyan)

[19]. Typically, gold fiducial markers are placed into the prostate target prior to simulation to aid in tracking during definitive radiation therapy and in some recurrent settings when a recurrent prostate bed nodule exists.

External beam radiation planning has evolved over time with increasing accuracy and decreased normal tissue exposure. Currently in the USA, intensity-modulated radiation therapy (IMRT) is the standard planning approach. IMRT allows for computer-optimized beam arrangements with modulated intensity resulting in more conformality than older 2D and 3D conformal radiation therapy (3DCRT) treatment approaches [13, 20, 21]. This conformality allows better sparing of nontarget tissues such as the bladder and bowel, which has been instrumental in optimizing outcomes by allowing safe dose escalation strategies. At Memorial Sloan Kettering Cancer Center, the 7-year late grade ≥2 and grade ≥3 GU toxicity was 21.1% and 2.2%, respectively, with dose escalation to 86.4 Gy in 1.8 cGy daily fractions, representing similar toxicity rates compared with lower doses [21].

As treatment conformality has improved, safe delivery of higher doses of radiation in fewer fractions, known as hypofractionation, has become more feasible. For prostate cancer, a radiobiologic prediction model of tumor cell sensitivity to fraction size known as alpha-beta ratio predicts better tumor cell kill with higher dose per fraction [6]. Several large-scale trials have compared moderately hypofractionated dose regimens, typically 60–72 Gy delivered in 2.4–3.4 Gy daily fractions, to standard fractionation regimens in the definitive setting, demonstrating similar efficacy and GU-related toxicity (Table 6.1) [15, 22–24]. The PROFIT trial was a

Table 6.1 A summary of trials using moderately hypofractionated regimens

Trial	Patients (*n*)	Arms	Primary endpoint	Late GU toxicity
PROFIT [15]	Intermediate-risk prostate cancer ($n = 1206$)	78 Gy at 2.0 Gy/fraction vs. 60 Gy at 3.0 Gy/fraction	5 year BPFS 85% in both arms	Maximum late GU toxicity of 2: 20% versus 19% (NS) Maximum late GU toxicity of 3: 2.0% versus 2.8% (NS)
CHHiP [24]	Localized prostate cancer (pT1b-T3aN0M0)	74 Gy at 2.0 Gy/fraction versus 60 Gy at 3.0 Gy/fraction versus 57 Gy at 3.0 Gy/fraction	5 year FFS 88.3% versus 90.6% versus 85.9% 60 Gy non-inferior to 74 Gy ($p = 0.0018$) 57 Gy not non-inferior to 74 Gy ($p = 0.48$)	Frequency of grade ≥2 late GU toxicity at 5 years: 9.1% versus 11.7% versus 6.6% (NS)
HYPRO [23]	Intermediate- and high-risk prostate cancer ($n = 820$)	78 Gy at 2.0 Gy/fraction versus 64.6 Gy at 3.4 Gy/fraction (3 fraction per week)	7-year RFS 67.6% versus 71.7% ($p = 0.52$)	Incidence of grade ≥2 GU toxicity at 3 years: 39% versus 41.3% ($p = 0.073$) Incidence of grade ≥3 GU toxicity at 3 years: 12.9% versus 19% ($p = 0.021$)
RTOG 0415 [22]	Low-risk prostate cancer ($n = 1092$)	70 Gy at 2.5 Gy/fraction versus 73.8 Gy at 1.8 Gy/fraction	5-year DFS non-inferiority: 85.3% versus 86.3% ($p < 0.001$)	Maximum late GU toxicity of 2: 20.5% versus 26.2% ($p = 0.009$) Maximum late GU toxicity of 3: 21% versus 3.5% ($p = 0.22$)

randomized, non-inferiority trial that included intermediate-risk prostate cancer patients comparing 78 Gy in 1.8 Gy fractions to 60 Gy in 20 fractions [15]. At a median follow-up of 6 years, the hypofractionated regimen was non-inferior to standard fractionation (5-year biochemical freedom from failure 85% in both arms). While acute toxicities were similar across trials, late urinary toxicity was statistically significantly increased for the moderately hypofractionated regimen in RTOG 0415 [22]. It is notable that the HYPRO trial was designed as a superiority trial to detect a 10% improvement in relapse-free survival in the moderately hypofractionated arm combined with a non-inferiority approach for toxicity, neither of which were confirmed in the results [22]. Taken together, moderately hypofractionated regimens appear similar in terms of outcome and toxicity and are largely replacing conventionally fractionated regimens, although do not yet have a long-term (>10–15-year) follow up.

Ultrahypofractionated radiation therapy (UH-RT), typically >4–10 Gy per fraction delivered either daily or every other day, has also become increasingly popular for both convenience and moderate-term data, suggesting its safety and efficacy. An example of a typical UH-RT plan is provided in Fig. 6.3. Overall, reported outcomes with UH-RT appear excellent. The Scandinavian HYPO-RT-PC trial was a randomized, non-inferiority trial comparing conventional fractionation (78 Gy in 39 daily

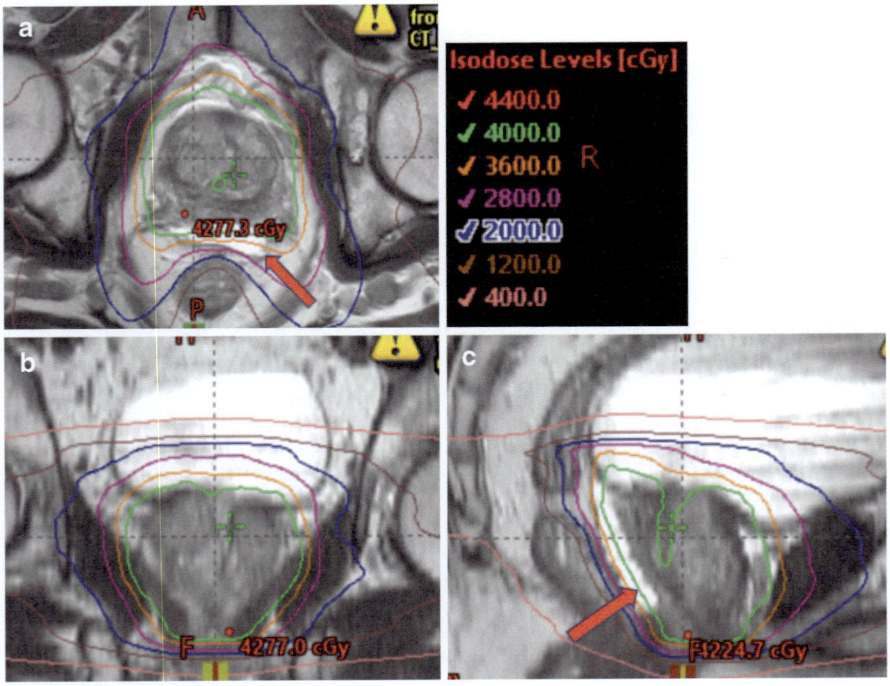

Fig. 6.3 (**a**–**c**) Axial (**a**), coronal (**b**), and sagittal (**c**) T2 MRI planning images for ultrahypofractionated RT (i.e., stereotactic body radiotherapy (SBRT)). Red arrow indicates rectal spacer. Green line = prescription (100%) isodose line

fractions) to UH-RT (42.7 Gy in 7 fractions delivered 3 days per week) for 1200 men with intermediate- to high-risk prostate cancer. No ADT was utilized. At a median follow-up of 5 years, both arms had a similar 5-year failure-free survival of 84% (95% CI, 80–87) with an adjusted HR of 1.002 (95% CI, 0.758–1.325; log rank, $p = 0.99$) [25]. While there was a modest increase in urinary toxicity in the UH-RT arm at 1-year follow-up (6 vs. 2%, $P = 0.0037$), there were no significant differences in late toxicity beyond 1 year [25]. The PACE-B trial included 874 low- and intermediate-risk men and similarly compared conventionally fractionated RT (78 Gy in 39 daily fractions) to UH-RT (36.25 Gy in 5 fractions over 1–2 weeks). RTOG grade 2 or higher GU toxicity was seen in 2 and 3% of patients in the conventionally fractionated arm and UH-RT arm, respectively, at 24 months ($p = 0.39$) [26].

In the postoperative setting, EBRT may be administered in patients who are at high risk of recurrence (i.e., positive margins, extracapsular extension, or seminal vesicle invasion) or in the salvage setting (i.e., persistently detectable or rising PSA) [27]. While the optimal timing of postoperative radiation therapy is unclear, many prefer an early salvage therapy approach as an adjuvant therapy has not been shown to be superior in prospective trials and could overtreat certain patients [7–9, 28]. The TROG RAVES trial was a phase III randomized trial including 333 prostatectomy patients with a PSA ≤ 0.10 and high-risk features defined as positive surgical margins, extraprostatic extension, or seminal vesicle invasion who were randomized to adjuvant EBRT or early salvage EBRT. Notably, there were significantly higher rates of grade ≥ 2 GU toxicity in the adjuvant arm compared with the salvage arm (70% vs. 54% ($p = 0.002$)). Both arms experienced high rates of erectile dysfunction (96% in the salvage arm and 98% in the adjuvant arm) [7]. The GETUG-AFU 17 trial compared adjuvant versus salvage radiation therapy in 424 men with pT3-4aNx-0 prostate cancer post-prostatectomy with positive surgical margins and found higher rates of late grade ≥ 2 GU toxicity in the adjuvant arm (27% vs. 7% ($p < 0.0001$)) [8]. Similarly, the RADICALS trial included 1396 men with at least one of the following risk factors after prostatectomy: pT3–4, Gleason score ≥ 7, positive margins, or preoperative PSA ≥ 10 and compared adjuvant to salvage radiation. They reported significantly worse grade 1–2 GU toxicities with adjuvant RT as compared to salvage RT at <2 years (early) and ≥ 2 years (late) time points. Toxicities included cystitis (early: 25% vs. 12%, $p < 0.0001$; late: 13% vs. 7%, $p < 0.0005$), hematuria (early: 11% vs. 4%, $p < 0.0001$; late: 12% vs. 4%, $p < 0.0001$), and urethral stricture (early: 6% vs. 3%, $p = 0.020$; late: 6% vs. 3% $p = 0.0025$). Self-reported urinary incontinence (graded 0–24, best to worst) was worse at 1 year for those in the adjuvant radiotherapy group (mean score 4.8 vs. 4.0, $p = 0{\cdot}0023$), but this difference did not persist at later time points [9]. It is worth noting that factors associated with incontinence in the postoperative RT setting include time elapsed from RP to initiation of RT, age, baseline incontinence levels, and radiation dose [29, 30].

An alternative to photon-based external beam radiation, proton therapy uses charged particles that provide some unique advantages in terms of dose distribution and radiobiology. Proton beam therapy has the physical property of traveling through tissues before slowing down and releasing energy at a prespecified depth. The release of energy, known as the Bragg peak, can be spread out to conform to a target's size/position with avoidance of "exit dose," a property of photon beam therapy that delivers low dose to nontarget tissue (integral dose). The clinical significance of this difference in integral dose between photon and proton therapies is of some debate, although certain clinical scenarios may warrant proton consideration such as patients at particular risk for secondary malignancy (i.e., pediatric patients). It is also important to note that the relative biological effectiveness (RBE), or the ratio of absorbed dose that produces the same biological effect of protons to photons, is assumed to be 1.1, and hence prescribed doses may vary between proton and photon therapies. It is unclear if the distinction of RBE between proton and photon therapies has any clinical value for prostate cancer.

Despite the theoretical benefit described above, clinical data demonstrating an advantage for protons in the treatment of prostate cancer is limited. A prospective comparison trial of proton beam therapy and photon therapy for men with prostate cancer is ongoing (COMPPARE NCT03561220). Several retrospective studies have been reported, which suggest similar GI, GU, or sexual toxicities between modalities [31–33]. One such cross-matched study by Fang et al. looked at 394 patients with localized prostate cancer receiving equivalent doses with either proton beam therapy or IMRT. There were no statistically significant differences between IMRT and proton beam therapy in terms of grade ≥2 acute (p = 0.36) or grade ≥2 late (p = 0.22) GU toxicities when adjusted for confounders and predictive factors [32]. Limitations in the availability and cost of proton therapy as well as the absence of data superiority data have limited its use.

Brachytherapy

Brachytherapy involves the transperineal placement of temporary (high-dose rate; Ir-192) or permanent (low-dose rate; I-125, Pd-103, or Cs-131) radiation sources directly into the prostate/seminal vesicles, typically aided by transrectal ultrasound guidance (Fig. 6.4). Both high-dose rate (HDR) and low-dose rate (LDR) brachytherapy can be used alone or, for patients with higher-risk features, in combination with external beam radiation therapy both to provide dose escalation and to encompass areas of extraprostatic extension and/or lymphatic coverage.

Acute urinary symptoms following brachytherapy, much like those seen with EBRT, are predominantly irritative and obstructive. Immediate post-procedure obstructive symptoms are often a consequence of needle trauma and edema. Patients with large-volume prostate glands and high baseline lower urinary tract symptoms may be at higher risk for acute urinary retention (AUR) requiring catheterization, which occurs in 5–15% of patients. Typically, this is short-lived, and most patients can void after 3–5 days. Incontinence is very uncommon in the immediate post-implant period and if present may represent overflow incontinence due to AUR.

Several efforts have been explored to reduce perioperative urinary morbidity following brachytherapy including the use of intraoperative or perioperative

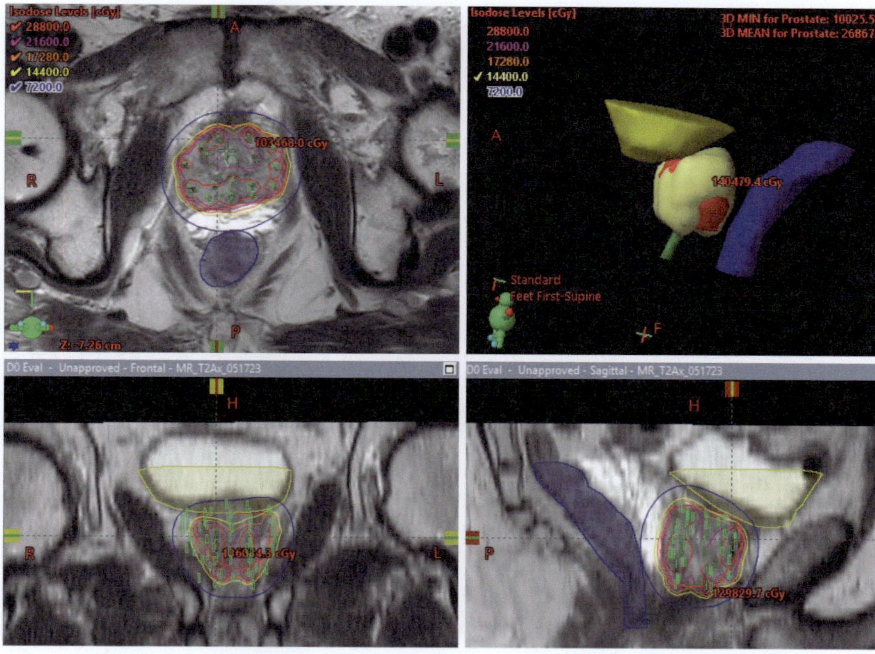

Fig. 6.4 An example of a typical low-dose rate (LDR) radioactive seed implant with rectal spacer in place

medication to counteract inflammatory effects. A prospective trial by Elshaikh et al. showed a significantly lower mean AUA score at 5 weeks after LDR in patients receiving perioperative tamsulosin, although there was no difference in urinary retention rates [34]. The use of perioperative corticosteroids is somewhat controversial with conflicting published data. A study published in 2003 showed that dexamethasone significantly reduced rates of urinary retention in patients undergoing LDR BT with or without EBRT [35]. Another more recent study found that LDR BT with perioperative prednisone yielded less severe worsening of EPIC urinary symptoms in the first month after treatment, although the effect was no longer evident at 3 months [36]. Conversely, in a randomized trial of men undergoing I-125 brachytherapy, intraoperative steroid used had no impact on urinary catheterization rate (1.5% in both arms) [37]. Similarly, the use of peri-procedure meloxicam did not reduce toxicity or urinary catheterization in a randomized trial of men undergoing prostate brachytherapy [38].

Acute urinary symptoms may be more pronounced with LDR compared with HDR, likely due to differing dose rates. A recent study from Memorial Sloan Kettering Cancer Center found a decreased incidence of grade 2 GU toxicity at 12 and 24 months in patients who had an HDR boost compared with an LDR boost with ultrahypofractionated RT (5 Gy in 5 fractions) (45% vs. 5.1% and 55% vs. 11%; $p < 0.001$) [39]. Similarly, Dhere et al. compared LDR and HDR boost and found a greater change in IPSS ($p = 0.003$) and EPIC-CP urinary score ($p = 0.002$)

in patients receiving LDR boost, with differences diminishing over time [40]. In general, most acute symptoms resolve by 3–6 months post-procedure. A phenomenon called a "urinary symptom flare" has been described following LDR, typically at 12–24 months post-implant and has been noted more commonly in patients with high baseline and maximal post-implant IPSS [41]. Late grade ≥3 toxicity, typically reported as urethral strictures or hemorrhagic cystitis, reportedly occurs in <5–8% of patients undergoing prostate brachytherapy [42–45]. The risk of urinary incontinence is <2% and often associated with post-radiation TURP [46].

For higher-risk patients, inclusion of periprostatic tissue and/or lymphatics may be necessary. Figure 6.5 demonstrates enhanced extraprostatic coverage with HDR. Providing dose escalation via a brachytherapy boost is particularly beneficial for reducing dose to normal adjacent tissue and providing direct dose escalation to intraprostatic targets. Three randomized trials comparing external beam radiation therapy with or without a boost have been reported [47–49]. The ASCENDE-RT trial included 398 men with intermediate- and high-risk prostate cancer to receive 12 months of ADT with 46 Gy to the pelvis and either an EBRT boost to 78 Gy or an LDR boost [47, 50]. At a median follow-up of 6.5 years, men undergoing EBRT alone were twice as likely to experience biochemical failure. In an analysis of toxicity, the cumulative incidence of grade 3 GU events was 18.4% in the LDR boost arm as compared to 5.2% in the EBRT alone arm ($P < 0.001$), although prevalence of grade 3 GU toxicity was lower (8.6% vs. 2.2%; $p = 0.58$) suggesting resolution [47, 50]. The most common type of GU event in this trial was urethral stricture requiring intervention which is notably higher than other reported series and may reflect technique and/or interventional propensity. Hoskin et al. reported a randomized trial comparing EBRT alone or EBRT with an HDR boost. In this trial, a 31% reduction in the risk of recurrence was noted in the HDR boost arm ($p = 0.01$) with similar incidence of late GU toxicity [48].

Several considerations are important in minimizing late toxicity related to brachytherapy-based approaches. During the brachytherapy planning process,

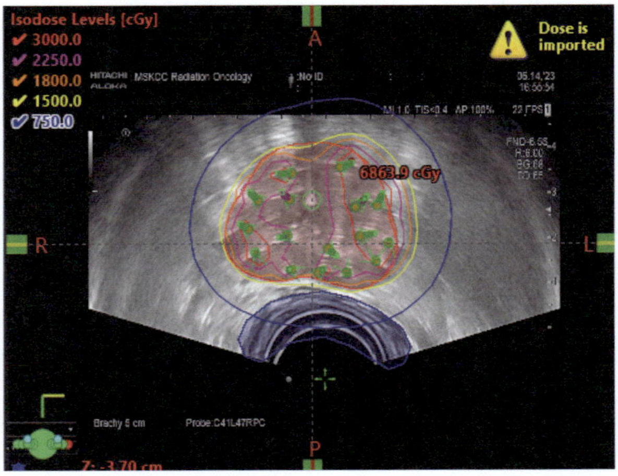

Fig. 6.5 HDR plan showing the increased coverage of the left anterolateral space in the patient with extraprostatic extension

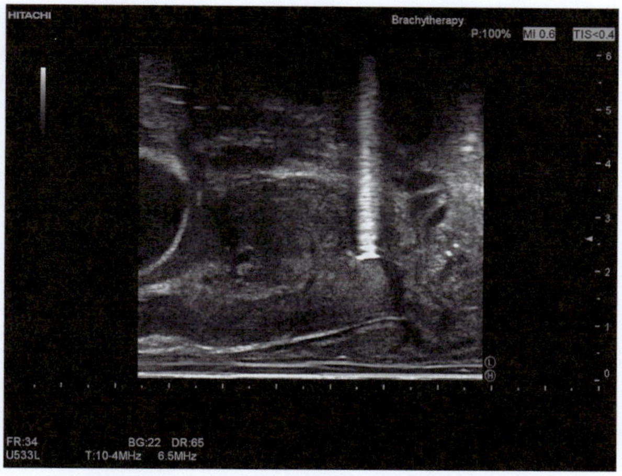

Fig. 6.6 Sagittal transrectal ultrasound image demonstrating the fiducial marker at the prostate apex

careful attention to the location of the genitourinary diaphragm on transrectal ultrasound and limitation of dose to this region is paramount. One approach is to place a fiducial marker at the prostate apex to ensure avoiding placement of seeds and/or HDR dose below this level (Fig. 6.6). Urethral doses have been weakly associated with urinary toxicity although the American Brachytherapy Society guidelines for both HDR and LDR exist [51, 52]. One German study found an association with urethral volume receiving ≥120% of the prescribed dose both significantly associated with late grade 3 GU toxicity [53]. Similar correlations of high urethral doses and urinary toxicity have also been reported [54]. In general, maintaining urethral doses <120% of prescription is advisable. Fibrotic tissue and telangiectasias post-radiation may be particularly prone to injury, and generally, interventions should be minimized to avoid worsened tissue damage. Urethral strictures should be managed with the least aggressive intervention possible to avoid post-intervention incontinence. Minor symptoms, such as transient hematuria, should resolve spontaneously, and after ruling out bladder lesions, hydration and briefly holding anticoagulants should suffice for treatment. More significant hematuria may be amenable to hyperbaric oxygen therapy before considering interventional approaches.

Sexual Functional Outcomes

Erectile dysfunction (ED) is a common complication of all prostate cancer therapies occurring in 50–80% of patients. Challenges to studying erectile outcomes include effects of aging, psychosocial factors, comorbidities, and concomitant medication effects. Additionally, definitions and assessment of erectile function vary across studies, leading to challenges in comparing results. Nevertheless, as an important quality of life concern for many patients, efforts to understand and modulate treatment effects are critical.

The exact pathophysiology of RT-induced ED is an area of active research. There have been multiple proposed mechanisms including those related to vascular, neurological, and endocrine dysfunction, and multifactorial mechanisms are most likely. Given that most patients with radiation-induced ED note declining function over time, late effects on vasculature likely dominate [55, 56]. Avoidance structures to reduce impact of radiation-induced ED proposed include the penile bulb, internal pudendal artery, corpora cavernosum, and neurovascular bundles [57, 58]. Prognostic factors for ED post-radiation include baseline erectile function, preexisting vasculopathy, neuropathies, and the use of androgen deprivation therapy [21, 59–61].

External Beam Radiation Therapy

Current guidance to limit effects of EBRT on erectile function include limitation of dose to periprostatic erectile structures including the penile bulb, proximal crura of the penis, and/or neurovascular structures. Visualization of the internal pudendal artery and neurovascular bundles is much more feasible with MRI-based planning. One phase II trial using vessel-sparing EBRT +/− brachytherapy and ADT suggested a favorable erectile preservation rate of 70.4% at 3 years and 66.7% at 5 years in men with baseline IIEF ≥16. Data from prospective trials suggest limiting dose to the penile bulb (perhaps as a surrogate for other relevant structures for erectile function) is also important [57, 62]. Additionally, in a study published by Thor et al., an association between maximum dose to the total penile structure defined as corpora cavernosa and penile bulb was the strongest predictor of ED symptoms [63].

As conformality of radiation dose to target tissues increases, effects on nontarget adjacent tissues are also reduced and may predict better toxicity profiles. A Japanese study comparing 3DCRT to IMRT found less impact on sexual function with the use of IMRT [64]. PACE-A, a randomized trial comparing UH-RT (36.25 Gy in 5 fractions) to radical prostatectomy for localized prostate cancer, reported better patient-reported sexual bother scores than the surgical cohort (abstract only) [65]. Ongoing trials examining erectile function-sparing EBRT are ongoing including POTEN-C (clinicaltrials.gov:NCT03525262) comparing standard with neurovascular-sparing CT-guided EBRT and ERECT trial (clinicaltrials.gov:NCT04861194) using neurovascular-sparing MRI-guided EBRT in a single-arm study.

Brachytherapy

The effect of brachytherapy on erectile function is dependent on whether it is used as a monotherapy or in combination with ADT and/or EBRT, with generally worse outcomes with combined therapies [66]. Theoretically, reduced radiation exposure to erectile structures is achievable with brachytherapy as compared to EBRT. Therefore, treatment with brachytherapy may lead to better erectile outcomes, particularly in younger men with optimal baseline function. Zelefsky et al.

reported similar erectile outcomes at 5 years in patients undergoing EBRT compared with LDR using I-125 (43% vs. 53% (ns)) [67]. Similarly, a large systematic review of erectile dysfunction post-radiation suggests similar ED rates among modalities [68]. In a study comparing Prostate Cancer Symptom Indices (PCSI) scores of baseline potent men undergoing RP, EBRT, BT, or active surveillance at 24 months, poor function was noted in 57.1% after RP, 27.2% after EBRT, 34.2% after brachytherapy, and 25.2% after active surveillance. For those with intermediate baseline function, 76.9% after prostatectomy, 55.0% after EBRT, 50.6% after BT, and 45.9% on active surveillance reported poor function at 24 months [69]. A prospective phase II trial of LDR for intermediate-risk localized prostate cancer found that rates of "moderate or big problem" with sexual function at 4 years was 29.7% as compared to 19.7% at baseline [70]. Hauswald et al. published 10-year results for patients receiving HDR monotherapy at UCLA from 1996 to 2009. Of the 448 patients, 70% were able to have erections suitable for intercourse at baseline. At median follow-up of 6 years, 225 patients were available for sexual function analysis of which 60% reported ability to have intercourse [45]. Further attempts to improve erectile outcomes may be feasible with focal brachytherapy approaches.

Increasingly, preventative strategies, aside from organ-sparing approaches, to improve erectile function posttreatment are being explored. Early initiation of PDE5 inhibitors, which induce smooth muscle relaxation in the corpus cavernosum and increase blood flow to the penis, post-prostatectomy has been shown to improve erectile recovery [71]. As the mechanism of erectile injury likely includes vascular effects, the potential for prophylactic use of PDE5 inhibitors to reduce RT-induced ED is of interest, but results have been mixed. RTOG 0831 was a randomized controlled trial evaluating patients undergoing both EBRT and brachytherapy alone who were randomized to tadalafil 5 mg daily for 6 months or placebo [72]. The primary outcome was a single IIEF question at 30 weeks, and no significant difference was noted between arms. In a more recent randomized prospective study by Zelefsky et al., daily sildenafil initiated 3 days pre-RT and continued for 6 months resulted in improved overall sexual function as measured by IIEF overall satisfaction as compared to placebo for all time points post-RT. Erectile function IIEF scores were significantly improved at 12 months, but no longer significant at 24 months for the sildenafil cohort [73]. A third randomized trial by Ilic et al. using prophylactic sildenafil for 6 months, beginning 1 month after completion of RT, showed better IIEF-5 scores at 4 weeks and 6 months that were not sustained over longer time periods [74]. This difference compared with the prior study by Zelefsky et al. may be attributed to the later initiation of the sildenafil, although further work is needed to understand the optimal use of prophylactic PDE5 inhibition including optimal agent, dosage, timing and duration of therapy.

Comparison of Treatment Modalities

Comparing toxicities of external beam radiotherapy, brachytherapy, and radical prostatectomy is challenging. Two large prospective studies have been published comparing patient-reported quality of life (QOL) outcomes for those who undergo surgery or radiation for their prostate cancer [59, 75]. The PROST-QA study [59] collected patient- and partner-reported outcomes before and after RP, EBRT +/− ADT, or LDR brachytherapy +/− EBRT for localized prostate cancer. Each treatment was associated with a different pattern of change in QOL domains of urinary, sexual, hormonal, and bowel function. Generally, RP was associated with worse initial sexual and urinary incontinence score, EBRT had worse initial bowel/rectal score with quickly resolving urinary irritation, and BT had worse initial and more slowly resolving urinary irritation. The use of hormone therapy worsened the adverse effects of EBRT or brachytherapy.

The ProtecT trial [75] compared men undergoing active monitoring, RP, or EBRT with hormone therapy. The 10-year outcomes of the combination of both cohorts showed evidence of substantial and persistent elevations in the rates of urinary incontinence (55% reported daily pad use at 6 months, reducing to 20% after 3 years and remaining stable thereafter) and ED (95% at 6 months, 85% at 6 years) following RP. For those undergoing RT, there was an increase in rates of nocturia (65% at 6 months, stabilized to 30–40% as was consistent with the other groups) and in the rates of ED (81.5% at 6 months, 70–72% at 6 years) and bloody stools (5% over 6 years).

Conclusion

Radiation therapy using brachytherapy-based treatment or external beam radiation therapy approaches is an effective therapy for prostate cancer. Imaging and treatment delivery technologies have evolved allowing radiation oncologists to better delineate structures, improve targeting, escalate dose to prostatic targets, and reduce dose to normal surrounding tissues. Future approaches include improving our understanding of radiation-induced mechanisms of injury, dose-effect relationships, and preventative strategies. Focal approaches using either BT or EBRT may allow further improvements on quality of life measures posttreatment in appropriately selected patients. Additionally, technological advances, including MR-based linear accelerators, may further improve targeting and adaptation of EBRT delivery with the potential to further decrease toxicity.

Take-Home Message

Radiation for prostate cancer is an established treatment that is mediated by free radical destruction of malignant cells. The collateral damage associated with radiation treatment is what mediates erectile dysfunction and irritative voiding symptoms and lower urinary tract symptoms. Patients should be counseled on the functional outcomes after radiation treatment. These are similar to post-prostatectomy outcomes in certain respects, but typically manifest over a longer period of time.

References

1. National Comprehensive Cancer Network. Prostate cancer [Internet]. 2023. [cited 2023 May 2]. Available from: https://www.nccn.org/professionals/physician_gls/pdf/prostate.pdf
2. Straub JM, New J, Hamilton CD, Lominska C, Shnayder Y, Thomas SM. Radiation-induced fibrosis: mechanisms and implications for therapy. J Cancer Res Clin Oncol. 2015;141(11):1985–94.
3. Kim JH, Jenrow KA, Brown SL. Mechanisms of radiation-induced normal tissue toxicity and implications for future clinical trials. Radiat Oncol J. 2014;32(3):103–15.
4. Riley PA. Free radicals in biology: oxidative stress and the effects of ionizing radiation. Int J Radiat Biol. 1994;65(1):27–33.
5. Travis EL. Organizational response of normal tissues to irradiation. Semin Radiat Oncol. 2001;11(3):184–96.
6. Hall EJ, Giaccia AJ. Radiobiology for the radiologist. 8th ed. Philadelphia: Wolters Kluwer; 2019. 597 p
7. Kneebone A, Fraser-Browne C, Duchesne GM, Fisher R, Frydenberg M, Herschtal A, et al. Adjuvant radiotherapy versus early salvage radiotherapy following radical prostatectomy (TROG 08.03/ANZUP RAVES): a randomised, controlled, phase 3, non-inferiority trial. Lancet Oncol. 2020;21(10):1331–40.
8. Sargos P, Chabaud S, Latorzeff I, Magné N, Benyoucef A, Supiot S, et al. Adjuvant radiotherapy versus early salvage radiotherapy plus short-term androgen deprivation therapy in men with localised prostate cancer after radical prostatectomy (GETUG-AFU 17): a randomised, phase 3 trial. Lancet Oncol. 2020;21(10):1341–52.
9. Parker CC, Clarke NW, Cook AD, Kynaston HG, Petersen PM, Catton C, et al. Timing of radiotherapy after radical prostatectomy (RADICALS-RT): a randomised, controlled phase 3 trial. Lancet. 2020;396(10260):1413–21.
10. Marshall DC, Kerns SL, West CML, Rosenstein BS. A comparison of radiation toxicity outcomes in patients with and without autoimmune diagnoses on the REQUITE study. Int J Radiat Oncol. 2021;111(3 Suppl):e238.
11. Shaikh PM, Singh SA, Alite F, Vargo JA, Emami B, Wu MJ, et al. Radiation toxicity in patients with collagen vascular disease: a meta-analysis of case-control studies. Int J Radiat Oncol Biol Phys. 2021;111(5):1214–26.
12. Hansen EK, Roach III M, editors. Handbook of evidence-based radiation oncology [internet]. Cham: Springer International Publishing; 2018 [cited 2023 Jul 5]. Available from: https://link.springer.com/10.1007/978-3-319-62642-0.
13. Michalski JM, Moughan J, Purdy J, Bosch W, Bruner DW, Bahary JP, et al. Effect of standard vs dose-escalated radiation therapy for patients with intermediate-risk prostate cancer: the NRG Oncology RTOG 0126 Randomized Clinical Trial. JAMA Oncol. 2018;4(6):e180039.
14. Kuban DA, Tucker SL, Dong L, Starkschall G, Huang EH, Cheung MR, et al. Long-term results of the M. D. Anderson randomized dose-escalation trial for prostate cancer. Int J Radiat Oncol Biol Phys. 2008;70(1):67–74.
15. Catton CN, Lukka H, Gu CS, Martin JM, Supiot S, Chung PWM, et al. Randomized trial of a hypofractionated radiation regimen for the treatment of localized prostate cancer. J Clin Oncol. 2017;35(17):1884–90.
16. Carrie C, Hasbini A, de Laroche G, Richaud P, Guerif S, Latorzeff I, et al. Salvage radiotherapy with or without short-term hormone therapy for rising prostate-specific antigen concentration after radical prostatectomy (GETUG-AFU 16): a randomised, multicentre, open-label phase 3 trial. Lancet Oncol. 2016;17(6):747–56.

17. Zaorsky NG, Shaikh T, Murphy CT, Hallman MA, Hayes SB, Sobczak ML, et al. Comparison of outcomes and toxicities among radiation therapy treatment options for prostate cancer. Cancer Treat Rev. 2016;48:50–60.
18. Widmark A, Klepp O, Solberg A, Damber JE, Angelsen A, Fransson P, et al. Endocrine treatment, with or without radiotherapy, in locally advanced prostate cancer (SPCG-7/SFUO-3): an open randomised phase III trial. Lancet. 2009;373(9660):301–8.
19. Hamstra DA, Mariados N, Sylvester J, Shah D, Karsh L, Hudes R, et al. Continued benefit to rectal separation for prostate radiation therapy: final results of a phase III trial. Int J Radiat Oncol Biol Phys. 2017;97(5):976–85.
20. Michalski JM, Yan Y, Watkins-Bruner D, Bosch WR, Winter K, Galvin JM, et al. Preliminary toxicity analysis of 3-dimensional conformal radiation therapy versus intensity modulated radiation therapy on the high-dose arm of the radiation therapy oncology group 0126 prostate cancer trial. Int J Radiat Oncol Biol Phys. 2013;87(5):932–8.
21. Spratt DE, Pei X, Yamada J, Kollmeier MA, Cox B, Zelefsky MJ. Long-term survival and toxicity in patients treated with high-dose intensity modulated radiation therapy for localized prostate cancer. Int J Radiat Oncol Biol Phys. 2013;85(3):686–92.
22. Lee WR, Dignam JJ, Amin MB, Bruner DW, Low D, Swanson GP, et al. Randomized phase III noninferiority study comparing two radiotherapy fractionation schedules in patients with low-risk prostate cancer. J Clin Oncol. 2016;34(20):2325–32.
23. Aluwini S, Pos F, Schimmel E, Krol S, van der Toorn PP, de Jager H, et al. Hypofractionated versus conventionally fractionated radiotherapy for patients with prostate cancer (HYPRO): late toxicity results from a randomised, non-inferiority, phase 3 trial. Lancet Oncol. 2016;17(4):464–74.
24. Dearnaley D, Syndikus I, Mossop H, Khoo V, Birtle A, Bloomfield D, et al. Conventional versus hypofractionated high-dose intensity-modulated radiotherapy for prostate cancer: 5-year outcomes of the randomised, non-inferiority, phase 3 CHHiP trial. Lancet Oncol. 2016;17(8):1047–60.
25. Widmark A, Gunnlaugsson A, Beckman L, Thellenberg-Karlsson C, Hoyer M, Lagerlund M, et al. Ultra-hypofractionated versus conventionally fractionated radiotherapy for prostate cancer: 5-year outcomes of the HYPO-RT-PC randomised, non-inferiority, phase 3 trial. Lancet. 2019;394(10196):385–95.
26. Brand DH, Tree AC, Ostler P, Voet H van der, Loblaw A, Chu W, et al. Intensity-modulated fractionated radiotherapy versus stereotactic body radiotherapy for prostate cancer (PACE-B): acute toxicity findings from an international, randomised, open-label, phase 3, non-inferiority trial. Lancet Oncol 2019;20(11):1531–1543.
27. Stephenson AJ, Scardino PT, Eastham JA, Bianco FJ Jr, Dotan ZA, Fearn PA, et al. Preoperative nomogram predicting the 10-year probability of prostate cancer recurrence after radical prostatectomy. JNCI J Natl Cancer Inst. 2006;98(10):715–7.
28. Vale CL, Fisher D, Kneebone A, Parker C, Pearse M, Richaud P, et al. Adjuvant or early salvage radiotherapy for the treatment of localised and locally advanced prostate cancer: a prospectively planned systematic review and meta-analysis of aggregate data. Lancet. 2020;396(10260):1422–31.
29. Bresolin A, Garibaldi E, Faiella A, Cante D, Vavassori V, Waskiewicz JM, et al. Predictors of 2-year incidence of patient-reported urinary incontinence after post-prostatectomy radiotherapy: evidence of dose and fractionation effects. Front Oncol [Internet] 2020 [cited 2023 Jul 17];10. Available from: https://www.frontiersin.org/articles/10.3389/fonc.2020.01207.
30. Munoz F, Sanguineti G, Bresolin A, Cante D, Vavassori V, Waskiewicz JM, et al. Predictors of patient-reported incontinence at adjuvant/salvage radiotherapy after prostatectomy: impact of time between surgery and radiotherapy. Cancer. 2021;13(13):3243.
31. Gray PJ, Paly JJ, Yeap BY, Sanda MG, Sandler HM, Michalski JM, et al. Patient-reported outcomes after 3-dimensional conformal, intensity-modulated, or proton beam radiotherapy for localized prostate cancer. Cancer. 2013;119(9):1729–35.

32. Fang P, Mick R, Deville C, Both S, Bekelman JE, Christodouleas JP, et al. A case-matched study of toxicity outcomes after proton therapy and intensity-modulated radiation therapy for prostate cancer. Cancer. 2015;121(7):1118–27.
33. Hoppe BS, Michalski JM, Mendenhall NP, Morris CG, Henderson RH, Nichols RC, et al. Comparative effectiveness study of patient-reported outcomes after proton therapy or intensity-modulated radiotherapy for prostate cancer. Cancer. 2014;120(7):1076–82.
34. Elshaikh MA, Ulchaker JC, Reddy CA, Angermeier KW, Klein EA, Chehade N, et al. Prophylactic tamsulosin (Flomax) in patients undergoing prostate 125I brachytherapy for prostate carcinoma: final report of a double-blind placebo-controlled randomized study. Int J Radiat Oncol Biol Phys. 2005;62(1):164–9.
35. Sacco DE, Daller M, Grocela JA, Babayan RK, Zietman AL. Corticosteroid use after prostate brachytherapy reduces the risk of acute urinary retention. BJU Int. 2003;91(4):345–9.
36. Keller A, Abdelhakiem M, Mulherkar R, Ghanta S, Benoit R, Smith RP, et al. Effect of short-term corticosteroid usage on acute urinary toxicity following Cs-131 prostate brachytherapy. Brachytherapy. 2022;21(4):468–74.
37. Mierzwa ML, Barrett WL, Redmond K, Shirazi R, Kastl A, Kumar N, et al. Randomized trial to assess the efficacy of intraoperative steroid use in decreasing acute urinary retention after transperineal radioactive iodine-125 implantation for prostate cancer. Cancer. 2008;113(9):2605–9.
38. Crook J, Patil N, Wallace K, Borg J, Zhou D, Ma C, et al. A phase III randomized trial of the timing of meloxicam with iodine-125 prostate brachytherapy. Int J Radiat Oncol Biol Phys. 2010;77(2):496–501.
39. Kollmeier MA, Gorovets D, Flynn J, McBride S, Brennan V, Beaudry J, et al. Combined brachytherapy and ultra-hypofractionated radiotherapy for intermediate-risk prostate cancer: comparison of toxicity outcomes using a high-dose-rate (HDR) versus low-dose-rate (LDR) brachytherapy boost. Brachytherapy. 2022;21(5):599–604.
40. Dhere VR, Fischer-Valuck BW, Goyal S, Liu Y, Morgan TM, Ghavidel E, et al. Patient-reported outcomes after low-dose-rate versus high-dose-rate brachytherapy boost in combination with external beam radiation for intermediate and high risk prostate cancer. Brachytherapy. 2021;20(6):1130–8.
41. Keyes M, Miller S, Moravan V, Pickles T, Liu M, Spadinger I, et al. Urinary symptom flare in 712 125I prostate brachytherapy patients: long-term follow-up. Int J Radiat Oncol Biol Phys. 2009;75(3):649–55.
42. Prestidge BR, Winter K, Sanda MG, Amin M, Bice WS, Michalski J, et al. Initial report of NRG oncology/RTOG 0232: a phase 3 study comparing combined external beam radiation and Transperineal interstitial permanent brachytherapy with brachytherapy alone for selected patients with intermediate-risk prostatic carcinoma. Int J Radiat Oncol. 2016;96(2):S4.
43. Kittel JA, Reddy CA, Smith KL, Stephans KL, Tendulkar RD, Ulchaker J, et al. Long-term efficacy and toxicity of low-dose-rate ^{125}I prostate brachytherapy as monotherapy in low-, intermediate-, and high-risk prostate cancer. Int J Radiat Oncol Biol Phys. 2015;92(4):884–93.
44. Yoshioka Y, Suzuki O, Isohashi F, Seo Y, Okubo H, Yamaguchi H, et al. High-dose-rate brachytherapy as monotherapy for intermediate- and high-risk prostate cancer: clinical results for a median 8-year follow-up. Int J Radiat Oncol Biol Phys. 2016;94(4):675–82.
45. Hauswald H, Kamrava MR, Fallon JM, Wang PC, Park SJ, Van T, et al. High-dose-rate monotherapy for localized prostate cancer: 10-year results. Int J Radiat Oncol Biol Phys. 2016;94(4):667–74.
46. Kollmeier MA, Stock RG, Cesaretti J, Stone NN. Urinary morbidity and incontinence following transurethral resection of the prostate after brachytherapy. J Urol. 2005;173(3):808–12.
47. Morris WJ, Tyldesley S, Rodda S, Halperin R, Pai H, McKenzie M, et al. Androgen suppression combined with elective nodal and dose escalated radiation therapy (the ASCENDE-RT trial): an analysis of survival endpoints for a randomized trial comparing a low-dose-rate brachytherapy boost to a dose-escalated external beam boost for high- and intermediate-risk prostate cancer. Int J Radiat Oncol Biol Phys. 2017;98(2):275–85.

48. Hoskin PJ, Rojas AM, Bownes PJ, Lowe GJ, Ostler PJ, Bryant L. Randomised trial of external beam radiotherapy alone or combined with high-dose-rate brachytherapy boost for localised prostate cancer. Radiother Oncol. 2012;103(2):217–22.
49. Moideen N, Crook JM, Araujo CD, Batchelar D, Castro F, Hilts M, et al. A randomized phase III trial comparing health-related quality of life after low dose rate (LDR) or high dose rate (HDR) prostate brachytherapy boost combined with external beam pelvic radiotherapy (EBRT). Int J Radiat Oncol Biol Phys. 2022;114(3):S3–4.
50. Rodda S, Tyldesley S, Morris WJ, Keyes M, Halperin R, Pai H, et al. ASCENDE-RT: an analysis of treatment-related morbidity for a randomized trial comparing a low-dose-rate brachytherapy boost with a dose-escalated external beam boost for high- and intermediate-risk prostate cancer. Int J Radiat Oncol Biol Phys. 2017;98(2):286–95.
51. Yamada Y, Rogers L, Demanes DJ, Morton G, Prestidge BR, Pouliot J, et al. American Brachytherapy Society consensus guidelines for high-dose-rate prostate brachytherapy. Brachytherapy. 2012;11(1):20–32.
52. King MT, Keyes M, Frank SJ, Crook JM, Butler WM, Rossi PJ, et al. Low dose rate brachytherapy for primary treatment of localized prostate cancer: a systemic review and executive summary of an evidence-based consensus statement. Brachytherapy. 2021;20(6):1114–29.
53. Ghadjar P, Oesch SL, Rentsch CA, Isaak B, Cihoric N, Manser P, et al. Late toxicity and five year outcomes after high-dose-rate brachytherapy as a monotherapy for localized prostate cancer. Radiat Oncol. 2014;9(1):122.
54. Ohashi T, Yorozu A, Saito S, Tanaka N, Katayama N, Kojima S, et al. Urinary and rectal toxicity profiles after permanent Iodine-125 implant brachytherapy in Japanese men: Nationwide J-POPS multi-institutional prospective cohort study. Int J Radiat Oncol Biol Phys. 2015;93(1):141–9.
55. Siglin J, Kubicek GJ, Leiby B, Valicenti RK. Time of decline in sexual function after external beam radiotherapy for prostate cancer. Int J Radiat Oncol Biol Phys. 2010;76(1):31–5.
56. Zelefsky MJ, Eid JF. Elucidating the etiology of erectile dysfunction after definitive therapy for prostatic cancer. Int J Radiat Oncol. 1998;40(1):129–33.
57. Roach M, Winter K, Michalski JM, Cox JD, Purdy JA, Bosch W, et al. Penile bulb dose and impotence after three-dimensional conformal radiotherapy for prostate cancer on RTOG 9406: findings from a prospective, multi-institutional, phase I/II dose-escalation study. Int J Radiat Oncol. 2004;60(5):1351–6.
58. McLaughlin PW, Troyer S, Berri S, Narayana V, Meirowitz A, Roberson PL, et al. Functional anatomy of the prostate: implications for treatment planning. Int J Radiat Oncol Biol Phys. 2005;63(2):479–91.
59. Sanda MG, Dunn RL, Michalski J, Sandler HM, Northouse L, Hembroff L, et al. Quality of life and satisfaction with outcome among prostate-cancer survivors. N Engl J Med. 2008;358(12):1250–61.
60. Alemozaffar M, Regan MM, Cooperberg MR, Wei JT, Michalski JM, Sandler HM, et al. Prediction of erectile function following treatment for prostate cancer. JAMA. 2011;306(11):1205–14.
61. Martell K, Bayley C, Quirk S, Braun J, Sun L, Smith W, et al. Predicting erectile dysfunction after highly conformal, hypofractionated radiotherapy to the prostate. Radiation. 2023;3(2):87–97.
62. Murray J, Gulliford S, Griffin C, Wilkins A, Syndikus I, Staffurth J, et al. Evaluation of erectile potency and radiation dose to the penile bulb using image guided radiotherapy in the CHHiP trial. Clin Transl Radiat Oncol. 2020;21:77–84.
63. Thor M, Olsson CE, Oh JH, Alsadius D, Pettersson N, Deasy JO, et al. Radiation dose to the penile structures and patient-reported sexual dysfunction in long-term prostate cancer survivors. J Sex Med. 2015;12(12):2388–97.
64. Namiki S, Ishidoya S, Tochigi T, Kawamura S, Kuwahara M, Terai A, et al. Health-related quality of life after intensity modulated radiation therapy for localized prostate cancer: comparison with conventional and conformal radiotherapy. Jpn J Clin Oncol. 2006;36(4):224–30.
65. Van As NJ, Tree A, Ostler PJ, van der Voet H, Ford D, Tolan S, et al. PACE-A: an international phase 3 randomised controlled trial (RCT) comparing stereotactic body radiotherapy (SBRT)

to surgery for localised prostate cancer (LPCa)—primary endpoint analysis. J Clin Oncol. 2023;41(6_suppl):298–298
66. Akbal C, Tinay İ, Şimşek F, Turkeri LN. Erectile dysfunction following radiotherapy and brachytherapy for prostate cancer: pathophysiology, prevention and treatment. Int Urol Nephrol. 2008;40(2):355–63.
67. Zelefsky MJ, Wallner KE, Ling CC, Raben A, Hollister T, Wolfe T, et al. Comparison of the 5-year outcome and morbidity of three-dimensional conformal radiotherapy versus transperineal permanent iodine-125 implantation for early-stage prostatic cancer. J Clin Oncol Off J Am Soc Clin Oncol. 1999;17(2):517–22.
68. Gaither TW, Awad MA, Osterberg EC, Murphy GP, Allen IE, Chang A, et al. The natural history of erectile dysfunction after prostatic radiotherapy: a systematic review and meta-analysis. J Sex Med. 2017;14(9):1071–8.
69. Chen RC, Basak R, Meyer AM, Kuo TM, Carpenter WR, Agans RP, et al. Association between choice of radical prostatectomy, external beam radiotherapy, brachytherapy, or active surveillance and patient-reported quality of life among men with localized prostate cancer. JAMA. 2017;317(11):1141–50.
70. Frank SJ, Pugh TJ, Blanchard P, Mahmood U, Graber WJ, Kudchadker RJ, et al. Prospective phase 2 trial of permanent seed implantation prostate brachytherapy for intermediate-risk localized prostate cancer: efficacy, toxicity, and quality of life outcomes. Int J Radiat Oncol Biol Phys. 2018;100(2):374–82.
71. Mulhall J, Land S, Parker M, Waters WB, Flanigan RC. The use of an erectogenic pharmacotherapy regimen following radical prostatectomy improves recovery of spontaneous erectile function. J Sex Med. 2005;2(4):532–40; discussion 540–2
72. Bruner D, Pugh SL, Pisansky TM, Greenberg RE, Pervez N, Reed DR, et al. Preliminary results of RTOG 0831, a randomized, double-blinded, placebo-controlled trial of tadalafil in the prevention of erectile dysfunction in patients treated with radiotherapy for prostate cancer. J Clin Oncol. 2013;31(15_suppl):9525.
73. Zelefsky MJ, Shasha D, Branco RD, Kollmeier M, Baser RE, Pei X, et al. Prophylactic sildenafil citrate improves select aspects of sexual function in men treated with radiotherapy for prostate cancer. J Urol. 2014;192(3):868–74.
74. Ilic D, Hindson B, Duchesne G, Millar JL. A randomised, double-blind, placebo-controlled trial of nightly sildenafil citrate to preserve erectile function after radiation treatment for prostate cancer. J Med Imaging Radiat Oncol. 2013;57(1):81–8.
75. Neal DE, Metcalfe C, Donovan JL, Lane JA, Davis M, Young GJ, et al. Ten-year mortality, disease progression, and treatment-related side effects in men with localised prostate cancer from the ProtecT randomised controlled trial according to treatment received. Eur Urol. 2020;77(3):320–30.

Trifecta Outcomes of Robot-Assisted Radical Prostatectomy: The "Balancing Act" of Achieving Cancer Control and Minimizing Collateral Damage

7

Prasanna Sooriakumaran, Harveer S. Dev, Erica Huang, Joshua Tran, Rafael Gevorkyan, Thomas E. Ahlering, and Peter Wiklund

Defining Biochemical Recurrence After Radical Prostatectomy

To this day, prostate cancer remains the most common nondermatological malignancy in Western men, with the vast majority of cases presenting with localized or locally advanced disease [1]. A standard treatment option for this is radical prostatectomy (RP), which was traditionally performed via the open approach, but more recently is typically conducted using robotic assistance (robotic-assisted radical prostatectomy (RARP)). As localized/locally advanced prostate cancer has a long natural history, studies examining survival take many years to mature and thus often suffer from low power. Hence, intermediate markers of oncologic outcome have become abundant in the literature, the most common being biochemical recurrence (BCR). This is defined as a rise in a prostate-specific, but not cancer-specific,

P. Sooriakumaran
University College London Hospital, London, UK

H. S. Dev
University of Cambridge, Department of Oncology, Cambridge, UK
e-mail: hsd26@cam.ac.uk

E. Huang · J. Tran · T. E. Ahlering (✉)
University of California, Irvine, Department of Urology, Irvine, CA, USA
e-mail: tahlerin@hs.uci.edu

R. Gevorkyan
Department of Urology, University of Southern California, Keck School of Medicine, Los Angeles, CA, USA
e-mail: rgevorky@usc.edu

P. Wiklund
Icahn School of Medicine at Mount Sinai, Department of Urology, New York, NY, USA
e-mail: peter.wiklund@mountsinai.org

S. Razdan, S. Razdan (eds.), *Urinary Continence and Sexual Function After Robotic Prostatectomy, Radiation, and Novel Therapies*,
https://doi.org/10.1007/978-3-031-64245-6_7

protein called prostate-specific antigen (PSA) released in the blood. While the exact rise that defines BCR is not universally agreed upon, most authorities use a PSA of 0.2 ng/mL or greater [2]. This threshold has been controversial as some argue that a PSA of 0.4 ng/mL or greater is a better predictor for further metastases [3].

Due to competing causes of mortality (more precisely the highly beneficial effects of ADT) in men with BCR post-RP, most recurrences do not lead to death. Thus, BCR is regarded as the initial metric, although not precisely predictive, of prostate cancer-specific mortality [4]. Moreover, it is the initial indicator of the need for salvage therapy [5]. The largest study examined 1997 men post-prostatectomy from 1982 to 1997, of which 15% developed BCR. Thirty-five percent of patients with BCR developed metastases after a median of 8 years, and 43% died of prostate cancer, after a median of circa 5 years after metastases [6, 7]. Hence, the risk of death from prostate cancer in those with BCR was 15%. A more recent study has quoted a 21% risk of death in men with BCR post-RP, and clearly, case mix is responsible for some of these differences [4]. Regardless, lethal metastatic disease is almost always preceded by a rise in PSA that signifies BCR.

How Positive Surgical Margins Correlate with Oncologic Outcome

A positive surgical margin (PSM) may reflect residual cancer cells at the edge of the surgical resection, and this is a consistent predictor of BCR [8–12]; one study reported a BCR-free survival of 93.8 and 79.9% after adjustment for covariates in those with negative and positive surgical margins, respectively [13]. A more recent study found that PSMs were only associated with BCR if there were multiple positive margins, ≥3 mm in length, or were composed of cancer with a Gleason score of 4 or higher [14]. Furthermore, studies directly comparing the effect of a PSM to metastasis-free survival and mortality are much less conclusive. A large registry study of 65,633 patients demonstrated a significant effect of PSM on cancer-specific mortality (HR, 1.70 [1.32–2.18]) [12]. However, criticism of this work has been directed at the absence of preoperative PSA data, and a recent audit that identified a significant rate of inaccurate coding in the database [15], although a second study has further supported the same conclusions from the SEER database, with PSM affecting mortality after multivariate modeling (HR, 1.4 [1.0–1.9]; $p = 0.036$) [9]. Nonetheless, some studies that have shown PSM to predict BCR have failed to demonstrate a significant relationship with mortality [8, 16, 17]. With such large differences in follow-up, inclusion criteria, and the accurate capture of covariates, it is unsurprising that the literature is conflicting as to whether PSM per se has a direct effect on prostate cancer mortality [18].

What we do know is that the vast majority of studies examining the relationship between PSM and oncologic outcome have done so after open RP. However, RARP has become the market leader in the United States and many other Western nations [19]. Hence, more recent work has sought to compare PSM rates across surgical approaches and to determine the impact on PSM in the RARP population. A meta-analysis based on 400 original articles used propensity score adjustments to demonstrate similar PSM rates for RARP and open RP [20], although a recent retrospective study of over 22,000 RP cases showed superior PSM rates in minimally invasive cases over open RP [21].

Multifocal Margins and Oncologic Outcome

If we accept some of the evidence cited earlier that PSM itself is associated with BCR, we might intuitively expect that multifocal tumors should be at greater risk for more residual tissue to be left behind and BCR to occur more quickly. To this end, a study of 210 men with PSMs revealed a 2.19-fold greater risk of recurrence in those with two or more PSMs compared to a unifocal margin [22]. Swanson et al. [23] described an overall crude (unadjusted) recurrence rate across seven recent large case series of 20 and 70% between unifocal and multifocal diseases. However, this result has not been reproduced by larger studies [24, 25], where the additional negative prognostic effect of an additional PSM has not been realized [26]. In a recent review of studies from 2005 to 2011, Fontenot [27] identified three studies where multifocality was found to confer a greater risk of BCR compared to unifocality [28–30], and seven in which no such additive effect was seen [8, 31–33].

The Impact of Margin Length

The impact of margin length would follow similar arguments to the impact of multifocality on BCR outcomes. However, most studies on PSM and BCR in both the open and robotic literature do not report on the PSM length and so we are limited to a few reports on which to draw our inferences. Furthermore, studies have generally reduced margin length into a categorical variable, often separating into <1/≥1 mm or < 3/≥3 mm. Noting the aforementioned, there have been four recent studies [34–37] that found an increasing PSM length to increase the risk of BCR, while three studies failed to show any significant increase in BCR risk on multivariable analyses [32, 38, 39].

Shikanov and colleagues demonstrated a relationship between the PSM length and risk of BCR in 1398 cases of RARP after a median follow-up of 1 year. They were unable to demonstrate an effect of PSM <1 mm on BCR and postulate that these may represent false-positive margins. However, an analysis of 294 RARPs with PSM, which reported margin length as a continuous variable, showed a correlation with BCR across all PSM lengths [34]. A more robust analysis of RARP patients with at least 5 years of follow-up established the predictive capability of PSMs ≥3 mm/multifocal margins compared to those <3 mm/unifocal margins (HR, 2.84 [1.76–4.59]), and this effect was even more substantial in lower-risk cohorts [40].

The Impact of Margin Location

So if the margin length is important in predicting oncologic outcome, the next question is whether the site of the PSM matters. If papers dealing with margin length were few and far between, this problem is even greater for the margin location literature, with most studies having insufficient power to pick up any association between margin location and BCR, especially after covariate adjustment or subgroup stratification. The subject is further complicated by inconsistent reporting methods of locations, with the International Society of Urological Pathologists and the College of American Pathologists proposing different classifications of PSM locations [27]. In general, the following are considered by most investigators to be appropriate descriptors for PSM location [27]:

1. *Apex*: The most distal aspect of the prostate is the most surgically challenging to access especially as we try to maximize the preserved urethral length. The prostatic apex passes adjacent to the dorsal venous complex and neurovascular bundles under the pubis [27]. It also presents difficulties during histopathologic analysis because of a sparse "capsule" which complicates correctly labeling PSMs as organ-confined tumors with an intraprostatic incision (pT2 with PSM), or a margin-positive extraprostatic tumor (pT3 with PSM), and risks incorrectly labeling organ-confined tumors (pT2 with negative margin, NSM). Hence, the PSM data at the apex is hugely subjected to the Will Rogers phenomenon in which both pT2 and pT3 PSM rates would be reduced if apical PSMs are reported as pT3 PSM cases due to a lack of a "capsule" [41]. The apex is considered to be the most common location for PSM across the ORP literature [42]. Although some studies showed a significantly increased risk of BCR with apical PSM after multivariable analysis, others have shown no such relationship [27]; the problem is that prostate cancer that reaches the apex may be indicative of larger tumor volume which may then confound multivariable analyses [43].
2. *Posterolateral and posterior*: Posterolateral margins are the second most common [42] and most often a result of efforts to preserve the neurovascular bundles, as this broadly describes the region where intra–/interfascial dissection occurs for nerve sparing. Three recent reports describe a greater impact on BCR rates with a PSM in this area, while only one failed to demonstrate a significant relationship (of any location including posterolateral) after multivariable regression, likely due to the small sample size [44]. Prostate cancers can also invade posteriorly into the Denonvilliers fascia necessitating resection of this posterior fascia. The association between PSM in this region and BCR has also been varied; Fontenot summarized three studies from the last decade which support both conclusions [27].
3. *Base and bladder neck*: The basal prostate refers to the cranial end of the prostate around the bladder neck, although PSMs at these sites are often grouped together [37]. PSM here can result from surgical efforts to preserve the bladder neck in an attempt to improve urinary continence recovery. The finding of an isolated PSM at the bladder neck is a reasonably infrequent occurrence

(compared to microscopic invasion of the bladder neck, pT3 disease which need not necessarily have an associated PSM). Controversy regarding the impact of PSMs at these sites also exists, particularly for those at the base. Hsu and colleagues reviewed 117 RP patients with positive margins and described a significant impact of bladder neck PSM on BCR (HR, 1.29 [1.0–1.67]; $p = 0.046$). In contrast, other studies refute the impact of a PSM at the bladder neck on BCR [31, 37, 45].

4. *Anterior*: This is generally considered as a fibromuscular stromal region that is less commonly associated with finding PSMs, with an incidence of 2–15%. Anterior PSM may be associated with transitional zone tumors and those among the "anterior horns," which are at risk of iatrogenic cautery when controlling the surrounding vasculature. This again illustrates the inverse relationship between minimizing collateral damage and PSM rates. The study by Hsu and colleagues also revealed an effect of anterior PSM on BCR (HR, 1.17 [1.02–1.33]; $p = 0.027$), possibly as a result of greater iatrogenic intraprostatic incision during vascular control. However, similar to other sites, there remains ambivalence regarding the effect a PSM at this site has on BCR [35, 37, 44, 46, 47].

Differences with the Robotic Approach (Space of Retzius, Hood Tech, MUL)

One might predict the operative differences of minimally invasive RP may result in a distinct pattern of PSM. A study of 538 patients described the most common PSM site to be in the apical region for ORP (54%) compared to the posterolateral region (54%) for laparoscopic RP [48]. Guillonneau reported similar findings with 50 and 30% at the apex and posterolateral regions, respectively, for their series of 1000 consecutive laparoscopic RP [49]. Similarly, Patel and colleagues reported on 1272 PSMs in 8095 RARP procedures and in agreement with earlier studies [50] found the apex and posterolateral sites to be the most common PSM locations (36 and 29%, respectively) [51]. The findings suggest unique technical challenges for intraoperative dissection which may reflect in differing locations of PSM for different surgical approaches.

Sooriakumaran et al. were unable to draw statistically significant conclusions regarding the effect of PSM location on BCR. Initial trends suggest PSM locations in RARP have different prognostic values when compared to ORP, where there is more widely (albeit not completely) accepted importance of posterolateral margins and relative equipoise regarding apical margins [40]. If the fourth arm superomedial traction applied in RARP during nerve sparing is responsible for significantly more intraprostatic incisions, which are considered to have less effect on BCR, then posterolateral margins in RARP should have less oncologic impact than in ORP series.

In order to investigate the impact of PSM parameters (length and location) on BCR after RARP, we conducted a tri-institutional, trans-Atlantic analysis on the topic [52]. Between January 2002 and May 2013, clinicopathologic data on RARP patients was prospectively collected across three participating centers (two USA, one Europe). Patients who had received RARP for cTI-3 prostate cancer and did not meet any of the following exclusion criteria were included in this study: not received adjuvant hormonal or radiation therapy, PSA had been recorded for at least 3 years post-RP, and the margin status (presence or absence) of the histopathologic specimen had been recorded. In total, 400 consecutive patients fulfilled these criteria and were included in this study.

With the growing popularity of different robotic approaches, new techniques have been introduced and popularized to improve early and overall continence and sexual function. For example, the Retzius-sparing technique has been growing in popularity, demonstrating higher rates of continence recovery with equivalent erectile function recovery. A meta-analysis of this technique compared to standard RARP found statistically significant higher rates of immediate continence recovery after catheter removal [53]. At 3, 6, and 12 months, continence recovery was shown to be higher but did not reach statistical significance. Four studies in the analysis found that there was equivalent erectile function recovery; however, this would need to be further explored before a definite statement can be made. While these outcomes highlight the benefits of the technique, a potential drawback is the higher rates of PSM. Statistically significant higher rates of PSM were observed in pT2 tumors, with >pT3 tumors generally being higher but not reaching significance. Despite the increase in PSM rates, there were no differences in BCR rates at 1 year when compared to a standard RARP.

Wagaskar et al. describe a "hood technique" performed on 300 patients that resulted in a high continence rate with low rates of PSM, thus achieving early continence without compromising PSM [54]. While this technique does not have very high rates of continence recovery 1 week after catheter removal, recovery rates seem to increase at a much quicker rate. This has been observed with an 83% recovery 1 month post-op.

Another popular technique is the preservation of the membranous urethral length (MUL). First described by Coakley et al., men with longer MUL had faster urinary continence recovery after open RARP [55]. Ko et al. found that there was an increase in continence recovery without impacting PSM rates [56]. In a systematic review and meta-analysis published in 2017, Mungovan et al. found that every extra millimeter of MUL resulted in a 9% greater chance of complete continence recovery [57].

Margin Positive Cases Have Worse Pathologic Stage, Grade, and Preoperative PSA

When comparing a PSM with negative margin cases, chi-squared differences revealed a higher preoperative PSA, smaller prostate volume, and higher stage and grade disease.

Thirty-seven percent of PSM cases went on to develop BCR compared with just 10% of negative margin cases.

Posterolateral and Apical Margins Are the Most Common Sites of Margin Positivity with Retzius, Hood, MUL, and All Other Approaches to RARP

Multifocal, posterolateral, and apical regions contributed to the greatest number of PSMs (27, 27, and 32%, respectively) and not unexpectedly the largest number of BCR among PSM cases. The highest level of BCR as a proportion was found at the base, with over half of all margins (19 of 35) producing BCR.

A Positive Margin Adversely Affects Outcome

On univariate binary logistic regression analysis, margin positivity at the base demonstrated a 10.2× greater risk of BCR, compared to the 3–4× odds ratio for the other locations. The effect however was lost on multivariate analysis, and similarly, institution, BMI, and age become nonsignificant when covariates are included. However, the odds for BCR with a PSM versus NSM remained prominent: OR, 3.1 c.f. OR, 4.2 for stage ≥pT3b c.f. OR, 1.3 for preoperative PSA.

A Positive Margin at Any Location Favors BCR

All margin locations had a significantly greater chance than negative margins of resulting in BCR, with a trend in odds ratios favoring anterior and apical margins as predictors of BCR compared to margins at the base or posterolaterally (odds ratios, 3.36, 3.27, 3.01, and 2.97, respectively).

PSM and Margin Length ≥3 mm Has a Greater Effect on BCR in Lower-Risk Cohorts

Multivariate Cox regression identified an instantaneous hazard ratio of 1.85 for PSM versus NSM leading to BCR. Stratification by pathologic stage (≤pT2 vs. ≥pT3) and Gleason grade (≤3 + 4 vs. ≥4 + 3) revealed a substantially greater impact of a PSM in lower-risk cohorts: 3.06 versus 1.58 and 2.35 versus 1.67, respectively (all $p < 0.001$). This holds true for margin length, with PSM ≥3 mm having almost double the effect of ≤3 mm on BCR in lower-risk cohorts compared to all risk cohorts taken together.

Apical Margins Are More Hazardous than Posterolateral Margins

Propensity-adjusted Cox regression analysis revealed significant hazard ratios across all margin locations. Although the magnitude of the instantaneous risk of BCR differs between statistical models, the trend for apical locations to show greater effects across these multivariable models was noteworthy, particularly when compared to posterolateral margins: 3.54 versus 2.837 (on propensity-adjusted Cox regression), 2.334 versus 1.685 (on multivariate Cox regression), and 3.272 versus 2.966 (on binary logistic model). Hence, apical margins appeared to have a greater hazard of BCR than posterolateral margins, after statistical analysis based on a common reference (NSM).

Impact of PSMs, Grade, pstage, and pN+ on Need for ADT Treatment and/or PCSM/MFS

Historically, PSM, GGG, pstage, and lymph node positivity (pN+) are well-known identifiers used to stratify risk in patients post-RP for secondary treatment, prostate cancer-specific mortality (PCSM), and metastases-free survival (MFS). Nomograms, many cited by guidelines (EAU & AUA), include GGG, PSM, pstage, pN+, seminal vesicle involvement, first PSA following RP, and time to BCR as the best identifiers for these risks [17, 58–61]. Evidently, there is no consensus on a nomogram for the best predictors of PCSM and BCR following RP. In addition, most of these predictors are static perioperative factors. In 2018, Bill-Axelson et al. reported on the 29-year outcomes of 347 men who underwent RP around 1990. In the highest GGG 4,5, only 50% of men had died of prostate cancer. This reinforces that even in "high-risk" men, patients often die with, and not from, prostate cancer. It is also well established that prostate cancer BCR is less mortal and aggressive with a longer course of survival compared to most other cancers [7] PSA doubling time (PSADT) was initially established as a potential predictor for cancer aggressiveness and clinical progression in 1997 [62, 63]. Thus, multiple studies and models have evaluated PSADT as a potential strong predictor for the need for treatment and PCSM [64–66]. PSADT kinetics is a snapshot of how the patient's disease is progressing after RP and is not primarily based on pathological outcomes at the time of surgery.

In 2020, a study by Matsumoto et al. stratified patients by PSADT and Gleason score. In this study, 431 patients with BCR were stratified into low- ($N = 240$; Gleason ≤ 7 and/or PSADT ≥ 6 months) and high-risk ($N = 191$; GG 8–10 and/or PSADT <6 months) groups. Most importantly, the low-risk group showed no difference in the 10-year Kaplan-Meier analysis of castrate-resistant prostate cancer (CRPC)-free survival and cancer-specific survival. Thus, the authors concluded that observation after BCR without salvage therapy is a viable option for low-risk patients [67]. According to current guidelines, patients should be treated with ADT/RT at BCR, with earlier intervention indicative of a better prognosis [2, 68]. However, there is evidence that there are cohorts of patients that have not experienced PCSM despite BCR. Matsumoto et al. indicated that observation after BCR may be possible without salvage therapy for low-risk patients (Gleason ≤7, PSADT ≥6 months) [67]. In fact, the European Association of Urology (EAU) makes a "weak" recommendation of watchful waiting for patients with PSADT > 12 months [68]. The issue lies in a strong algorithm for evaluating which patients under observation can continue to be watched and when to move the patient to treatment if need be.

Management of Low-Risk BCRs with Observation Using PSADT Kinetics

A major concern facing oncological management again swings back to oncological versus continence and sexual function outcomes. In short, if a positive margin has negligible long-term oncologic impact, the preservation of important patient outcomes arguably reigns supreme. Along the same line of reasoning, there is continuing and growing evidence that potentially as many as 30–40% of men with BCR can be carefully managed without treatment using PSADT kinetics. In 2005, we first described a group of BCR patients who were managed at the Long Beach VA without treatment based primarily on PSADT greater than 18 months [64].

In 2022, we subsequently published on our own cohort of 407 BCR patients, 136 of whom have not needed treatment at a median follow-up of 7.5 years (IQR, 3.9–10.7). The patient's "initial" PSADT is based on the first three to four PSAs after BCR (0.2 ng/mL, x2). After establishing an "initial" PSADT, a subsequent "pattern" develops where the doubling times either increase or decrease over time (usually 30+ months post-op). Men with rapidly decreasing PSADT were unstable typically with a rapidly rising PSA and were treated with ADT or RT/ADT, with a 10.7% 15-year PCSM and 18.5% 15-year overall mortality. In distinction, men with an increasing PSADT or slowly decreasing high "initial" PSADT were watched and had no PCSM, establishing that there is a cohort (~33%) who can be managed with active observation without secondary treatments (RT/ADT) [69]. In ROC analysis, AUC was 0.83, indicative of a strong predictor of no treatment [66]. Thus, while preoperative PSA, pGGG, pstage, and age are helpful in determining risk, PSADT and PSADT kinetics arguably are better prognostic factors for how the disease is proceeding after surgery and thus should be considered for monitoring patients post-RP for the need for treatment.

Discussion

Our study found that PSMs are associated with a greater risk of BCR after RARP compared to negative margins. This concurs with growing evidence across open and minimally invasive series [31, 51]. It is not surprising that some of this effect is by association, and we see PSM associated with other risk factors for BCR such as tumor grade and stage. We demonstrated the greater impact PSM carries on lower-risk (pT2 or Gleason ≤3 + 4 or both) prostate cancers after subgroup analysis. This probably reflects a relative balance with other more influential factors. Gleason grade and tumor stage probably have the largest impact on risk of BCR [51, 70, 71], although PSM remains the most important "surgically controllable" predictor of BCR. Indeed, the presence of a PSM is itself dependent on some of these factors, most notably the pathologic stage: incidence of PSM has been reported as 9% for pT2, 37% for pT3, and 50% for pT4 [72]. So, this is the crux of the issue: with high-grade and stage tumors, the biology of the disease drives the risk of BCR with margin status having little independent predictive value over and beyond the biological variables. However, with low-risk tumors in which biology is unlikely to lead to progression and or PCSM, the relative increased risk of relapse with a PSM compared with a negative margin is greater. A report on nearly 1000 cases from the Karolinska University Hospital (Stockholm, Sweden) on men with at least 5 years of follow-up post-RARP confirms these findings [73].

The counterpoint of this argument is that the absolute risk of BCR is much higher for high-grade and stage tumors than for low ones, and thus any increased risk of relapse may be considered to be more important for the former cases. As our experience progresses with the oncologic perspective, it might thus be more imperative for the surgeon to attempt to get a negative margin at the cost of increasing collateral damage in these high-risk cases and be less concerned with getting negative margins in cases of low Gleason grade or stage. Here, the surgeon might choose to accept higher PSM for minimizing collateral damage and thus optimizing the functional outcomes of urinary continence recovery and erectile function. This is the balancing act that becomes the surgeon's edict. With nerve sparing during RARP most likely to lead to PSM in the posterolateral region, and our work described herein that suggests this has minimal impact on BCR, surgeons should not shy away from aggressive nerve sparing for low-risk RARP cases. This is even more important given recent data that the more aggressive the nerve sparing, the better the continence and erectile outcomes are [74].

Hazard ratios from our statistical modeling appear to suggest a weaker impact of posterolateral margins on BCR compared to other sites, and this is particularly surprising when compared to evidence from open RP, where the impact of posterolateral PSM on BCR is well established [42]. Indeed, Vickers and colleagues have described posterolateral PSM in pT2 disease as an adverse factor on outcome and related to inadequate surgical technique [75].

The lack of tactile feedback that results from operating with a robotic platform has long been cited as a potential reason for greater iatrogenic PSM. However, many have reported the use of visual cues to offset any loss in tactile feedback, and comparing crude PSM rates between studies seems to suggest fewer may be caused by robotic compared to open operations [76, 77]. That said, one hypothesis regarding posterolateral margins is the fourth arm robotic traction placed on the prostatic "capsule" and surrounding structures, particularly during craniomedial elevation of the vasa/seminal vesicles during posterolateral dissection. The sustained tension resulting from hitching up the prostate, particularly during prolonged periods when performing nerve sparing, is likely to facilitate easier dissection but perhaps also causes iatrogenic intraprostatic incisions. Secin and colleagues found a counterintuitive relationship between PSM and extrafascial nerve-sparing procedure, possibly resulting from a technical error forcing false planes and producing capsular flaps [18], although we did not have the "nerve-sparing" status as a variable for our analysis.

In a study of 2442 patients, Eastham and colleagues describe a significant impact of posterolateral margin status on BCR (HR, 2.8 [1.76–4.44]), but failed to demonstrate an effect of apical margins (HR, 0.94 [0.59–1.51]). Eastham comments on a higher risk of BCR in open RP series with posterolateral margins. as the area least likely to receive iatrogenic trauma as well as its proximity to nerves which permits perineural invasion [78]. They instead suggest the apex is under greater traction with false-positive margins, less supporting tissue at the apex providing less vascular support for metastatic spread [78]. While this cannot be discounted, this likely reflects the open surgical technique. Clearly, targeted traction of the robotic instruments around the prostate to facilitate nerve sparing can still cause iatrogenic damage while sparing the neurovasculature from direct injury.

Pettus and Pfitzenmaier have described a significant impact of apical PSM on BCR [11, 26], although Pettus's analysis fails on multivariate analysis; several other earlier studies including one of 172 patients over 3.5 years of follow-up also failed to demonstrate an association between apical PSMs and clinical progression [79, 80].

The findings of our study suggest apical margins are more hazardous than posterolateral ones in RARP and support a trend seen in one recent study [40]. While the apex has been shown to impact BCR in some studies from the ORP series, this effect is often less than a PSM elsewhere. While our study did not directly compare ORP and RARP cases, the dominance of apical margin positivity associated with BCR has not been seen before in the RARP series, and technical differences between the two surgical approaches must be considered at least partially responsible. Intraoperative differences in terms of approach, traction, and risk of iatrogenic capsular incisions are likely to be responsible for these differences.

Two of the three institutions involved in our multi-institutional study have made specific efforts toward altering their control of the dorsal venous complex prior to attempting apical dissection. Theories as to why the order of these two operative steps may affect apical PSM rates include the possible effect of bunching up tissues around the apex and distorting apical anatomy. Alternative methods (supported by the third institution of our study) advocate division of these vessels prior to apical dissection which would encourage more inferior incisions in an effort to avoid the dorsal veins and blood loss, which might inadvertently lead to an intraprostatic incision [40, 81, 82]. The apex is a technically challenging region to operate in, particularly with variations in shape. Technical modifications however continue to improve PSM rates, particularly at the apex, with variations in the RARP technique, e.g., retroapical approach [76], allowing better circumferential visualization of the apex and membranous urethra, leading to a total decrease as well as proportionally fewer apical margins as a percentage of total PSM burden. Because of these efforts, it should therefore follow that the PSMs that will remain at the apex are biologically rather than surgically attributable PSMs (i.e., fewer false positives) which would thus carry a worse prognosis.

Ergo, there are fewer apical margins evident with this technique, due to less false-negative iatrogenic damage to the apex. Although there were 27.5% margins classified as apical in our study, we do not have an open RP arm to compare with, and comparisons in the context of such a wide range of values in the literature are unhelpful. However, it remains possible that this reflects an increasingly smaller percentage of false-positive margins as a result of improved technical dissection using the robotic platform.

A failure to identify capsular incisions from pT3 PSM at the apex would falsely upstage the disease (Will Rogers phenomenon) and also lead to a lower-than-expected impact of the apical margin location when taking into account other variables in multivariable models. If carcinoma extends to the inked margin adjacent to benign prostatic glands, and in the absence of adipocytes, this can be used to differentiate PSM at the apex with associated extraprostatic extension (EPE). However, there is no consensus as to a reliable method to make this distinction, and many authors do not routinely diagnose EPE at the apex for this reason [83].

Understaging can also result from a phenomenon of fibrotic desmoplastic reaction following extraprostatic extension and can confuse any assessment of margin status, and this may lead to ascribing more importance to apical margins, although suggestions have been made that this occurs in the posterolateral region, which would further strengthen our findings of a difference between these locations [42].

We generally found higher hazard ratios associated with anterior and apical margins compared to posterolateral and basal ones, although the numbers involved at these sites were smaller. The anterior prostate is predominantly fibromuscular stroma, and a PSM here may reflect the inherent aggressiveness of any tumor able to migrate into it (rather than necessarily reflecting a site of origin that is innately aggressive—see earlier). It is also possible the close proximity to vasculature provides a more favorable location for distant spread.

Suggestions for future approaches to prevent PSM, beyond technical modifications, have included routine intraoperative frozen sections to permit secondary resection intraoperatively; 25% of cases are found to detect residual cancer on attempts at removing further tissue, implying a PSM may not always reflect residual cancer in the prostatic bed [84]. Follow-up data is lacking regarding the effect on outcomes such as BCR rates in those treated using this method.

Conclusions

PSMs remain a critical finding to identify and better understand, given their profound patient implications in terms of prognosis and further treatment. All PSMs resulting from RARP are not equivalent; longer margins suggest a higher risk of recurrence and the influence is especially prominent in lower-risk patients. The apex is a significant contributor to BCR and appears to have the strongest impact of all the margin locations in RARP patients. In contrast, the posterolateral region appears to carry a smaller effect on BCR, probably reflecting greater iatrogenic injury to the prostate in this region. Hence, RARP surgeons might choose to accept the increased risk of posterolateral margins during nerve sparing in lower grade and stage prostate cancer patients, but rather make a wider dissection in the higher-risk cases sacrificing functional outcomes for lower PSM in these men.

Take-Home Message

The radical prostatectomy trifecta is to achieve cancer control, recover urinary continence, and recover erectile function. This chapter devotes time to discuss the razor's edge of positive surgical margin status at both prostate apex and posterolateral edges, with the desire of maximizing both the membranous urethral length and nerve sparing. These are the difficult decisions that must be made preoperatively and intraoperatively by the surgeon. As the authors duly noted, oftentimes the underlying pathology and risk status of the patient's disease will dictate the degree of dissection around the prostate.

References

1. Orr DP, Fineberg NS, Gray DL. Glycemic control and transfer of health care among adolescents with insulin dependent diabetes mellitus. J Adolesc Health. 1996;18(1):44–7.
2. Lowrance WT, Breau RH, Chou R, Chapin BF, Crispino T, Dreicer R, et al. Advanced prostate cancer: AUA/ASTRO/SUO guideline PART I. J Urol. 2021;205(1):14–21.
3. Amling CL, Bergstralh EJ, Blute ML, Slezak JM, Zincke H. Defining prostate specific antigen progression after radical prostatectomy: what is the most appropriate cut point? J Urol. 2001;165(4):1146–51.
4. Antonarakis ES, Chen Y, Elsamanoudi SI, Brassell SA, Da Rocha MV, Eisenberger MA, et al. Long-term overall survival and metastasis-free survival for men with prostate-specific antigen-recurrent prostate cancer after prostatectomy: analysis of the Center for Prostate Disease Research National Database. BJU Int. 2011;108(3):378–85.
5. Kim M, Yoo D, Pyo J, Cho W. Clinicopathological significances of positive surgical resection margin after radical prostatectomy for prostatic cancers: a meta-analysis. Medicina (Kaunas). 2022;58(9):1251.
6. Freedland SJ, Humphreys EB, Mangold LA, Eisenberger M, Dorey FJ, Walsh PC, et al. Risk of prostate cancer-specific mortality following biochemical recurrence after radical prostatectomy. JAMA. 2005;294(4):433–9.
7. Bill-Axelson A, Holmberg L, Garmo H, Taari K, Busch C, Nordling S, et al. Radical prostatectomy or watchful waiting in prostate cancer – 29-year follow-up. N Engl J Med. 2018;379(24):2319–29.
8. Boorjian SA, Karnes RJ, Crispen PL, Carlson RE, Rangel LJ, Bergstralh EJ, et al. The impact of positive surgical margins on mortality following radical prostatectomy during the prostate specific antigen era. J Urol. 2010;183(3):1003–9.
9. Chalfin HJ, Dinizo M, Trock BJ, Feng Z, Partin AW, Walsh PC, et al. Impact of surgical margin status on prostate-cancer-specific mortality. BJU Int. 2012;110(11):1684–9.
10. Mauermann J, Fradet V, Lacombe L, Dujardin T, Tiguert R, Tetu B, et al. The impact of solitary and multiple positive surgical margins on hard clinical end points in 1712 adjuvant treatment-naive pT2-4 N0 radical prostatectomy patients. Eur Urol. 2013;64(1):19–25.
11. Pfitzenmaier J, Pahernik S, Tremmel T, Haferkamp A, Buse S, Hohenfellner M. Positive surgical margins after radical prostatectomy: do they have an impact on biochemical or clinical progression? BJU Int. 2008;102(10):1413–8.

12. Wright JL, Dalkin BL, True LD, Ellis WJ, Stanford JL, Lange PH, et al. Positive surgical margins at radical prostatectomy predict prostate cancer specific mortality. J Urol. 2010;183(6):2213–8.
13. Alkhateeb S, Alibhai S, Fleshner N, Finelli A, Jewett M, Zlotta A, et al. Impact of positive surgical margins after radical prostatectomy differs by disease risk group. J Urol. 2010;183(1):145–50.
14. Lee W, Lim B, Kyung YS, Kim CS. Impact of positive surgical margin on biochemical recurrence in localized prostate cancer. Prostate Int. 2021;9(3):151–6.
15. Shah SK, Fleet TM, Williams V, Smith AY, Skipper B, Wiggins C. SEER coding standards result in underestimation of positive surgical margin incidence at radical prostatectomy: results of a systematic audit. J Urol. 2011;186(3):855–9.
16. Stephenson AJ, Eggener SE, Hernandez AV, Klein EA, Kattan MW, Wood DP, et al. Do margins matter? The influence of positive surgical margins on prostate cancer-specific mortality. Eur Urol. 2014;65(4):675–80.
17. Eggener SE, Scardino PT, Walsh PC, Han M, Partin AW, Trock BJ, et al. Predicting 15-year prostate cancer specific mortality after radical prostatectomy. J Urol. 2011;185(3):869–75.
18. Yossepowitch O, Briganti A, Eastham JA, Epstein J, Graefen M, Montironi R, et al. Positive surgical margins after radical prostatectomy: a systematic review and contemporary update. Eur Urol. 2014;65(2):303–13.
19. Trinh QD, Sammon J, Sun M, Ravi P, Ghani KR, Bianchi M, et al. Perioperative outcomes of robot-assisted radical prostatectomy compared with open radical prostatectomy: results from the nationwide inpatient sample. Eur Urol. 2012;61(4):679–85.
20. Tewari A, Sooriakumaran P, Bloch DA, Seshadri-Kreaden U, Hebert AE, Wiklund P. Positive surgical margin and perioperative complication rates of primary surgical treatments for prostate cancer: a systematic review and meta-analysis comparing retropubic, laparoscopic, and robotic prostatectomy. Eur Urol. 2012;62(1):1–15.
21. Sooriakumaran P, John M, Wiklund P, Lee D, Nilsson A, Tewari AK. Learning curve for robotic assisted laparoscopic prostatectomy: a multi-institutional study of 3794 patients. Minerva Urol Nefrol. 2011;63(3):191–8.
22. Sofer M, Hamilton-Nelson KL, Civantos F, Soloway MS. Positive surgical margins after radical retropubic prostatectomy: the influence of site and number on progression. J Urol. 2002;167(6):2453–6.
23. Swanson GP, Lerner SP. Positive margins after radical prostatectomy: implications for failure and role of adjuvant treatment. Urol Oncol. 2013;31(5):531–41.
24. Kausik SJ, Blute ML, Sebo TJ, Leibovich BC, Bergstralh EJ, Slezak J, et al. Prognostic significance of positive surgical margins in patients with extraprostatic carcinoma after radical prostatectomy. Cancer. 2002;95(6):1215–9.
25. Grossfeld GD, Chang JJ, Broering JM, Miller DP, Yu J, Flanders SC, et al. Impact of positive surgical margins on prostate cancer recurrence and the use of secondary cancer treatment: data from the CaPSURE database. J Urol. 2000;163(4):1171–7. quiz 1295
26. Pettus JA, Weight CJ, Thompson CJ, Middleton RG, Stephenson RA. Biochemical failure in men following radical retropubic prostatectomy: impact of surgical margin status and location. J Urol. 2004;172(1):129–32.
27. Fontenot PA, Mansour AM. Reporting positive surgical margins after radical prostatectomy: time for standardization. BJU Int. 2013;111(8):E290–9.
28. Stephenson AJ, Wood DP, Kattan MW, Klein EA, Scardino PT, Eastham JA, et al. Location, extent and number of positive surgical margins do not improve accuracy of predicting prostate cancer recurrence after radical prostatectomy. J Urol. 2009;182(4):1357–63.
29. Resnick MJ, Canter DJ, Guzzo TJ, Magerfleisch L, Tomaszewski JE, Brucker BM, et al. Defining pathological variables to predict biochemical failure in patients with positive surgical margins at radical prostatectomy: implications for adjuvant radiotherapy. BJU Int. 2010;105(10):1377–80.
30. Kordan Y, Salem S, Chang SS, Clark PE, Cookson MS, Davis R, et al. Impact of positive apical surgical margins on likelihood of biochemical recurrence after radical prostatectomy. J Urol. 2009;182(6):2695–701.

31. Shikanov S, Song J, Royce C, Al-Ahmadie H, Zorn K, Steinberg G, et al. Length of positive surgical margin after radical prostatectomy as a predictor of biochemical recurrence. J Urol. 2009;182(1):139–44.
32. May M, Brookman-May S, Weißbach L, Herbst H, Gilfrich C, Papadopoulos T, et al. Solitary and small (≤3 mm) apical positive surgical margins are related to biochemical recurrence after radical prostatectomy. Int J Urol. 2011;18(4):282–9.
33. Budäus L, Isbarn H, Eichelberg C, Lughezzani G, Sun M, Perrotte P, et al. Biochemical recurrence after radical prostatectomy: multiplicative interaction between surgical margin status and pathological stage. J Urol. 2010;184(4):1341–6.
34. Cao D, Humphrey PA, Gao F, Tao Y, Kibel AS. Ability of linear length of positive margin in radical prostatectomy specimens to predict biochemical recurrence. Urology. 2011;77(6):1409–14.
35. Hsu M, Chang SL, Ferrari M, Nolley R, Presti JC, Brooks JD. Length of site-specific positive surgical margins as a risk factor for biochemical recurrence following radical prostatectomy. Int J Urol. 2011;18(4):272–9.
36. Brimo F, Partin AW, Epstein JI. Tumor grade at margins of resection in radical prostatectomy specimens is an independent predictor of prognosis. Urology. 2010;76(5):1206–9.
37. Savdie R, Horvath LG, Benito RP, Rasiah KK, Haynes AM, Chatfield M, et al. High Gleason grade carcinoma at a positive surgical margin predicts biochemical failure after radical prostatectomy and may guide adjuvant radiotherapy. BJU Int. 2012;109(12):1794–800.
38. Psutka SP, Feldman AS, Rodin D, Olumi AF, Wu CL, McDougal WS. Men with organ-confined prostate cancer and positive surgical margins develop biochemical failure at a similar rate to men with extracapsular extension. Urology. 2011;78(1):121–5.
39. Marks RA, Koch MO, Lopez-Beltran A, Montironi R, Juliar BE, Cheng L. The relationship between the extent of surgical margin positivity and prostate specific antigen recurrence in radical prostatectomy specimens. Hum Pathol. 2007;38(8):1207–11.
40. Sooriakumaran P, Ploumidis A, Nyberg T, Olsson M, Akre O, Haendler L, et al. The impact of length and location of positive margins in predicting biochemical recurrence after robot-assisted radical prostatectomy with a minimum follow-up of 5 years. BJU Int. 2015;115(1):106–13.
41. Gofrit ON, Zorn KC, Steinberg GD, Zagaja GP, Shalhav AL. The Will Rogers phenomenon in urological oncology. J Urol. 2008;179(1):28–33.
42. Meeks JJ, Eastham JA. Radical prostatectomy: positive surgical margins matter. Urol Oncol. 2013;31(7):974–9.
43. Ohori M, Abbas F, Wheeler TM, Kattan MW, Scardino PT, Lerner SP. Pathological features and prognostic significance of prostate cancer in the apical section determined by whole mount histology. J Urol. 1999;161(2):500–4.
44. Saether T, Sørlien LT, Viset T, Lydersen S, Angelsen A. Are positive surgical margins in radical prostatectomy specimens an independent prognostic marker? Scand J Urol Nephrol. 2008;42(6):514–21.
45. Anastasiou I, Tyritzis SI, Adamakis I, Mitropoulos D, Stravodimos KG, Katafigiotis I, et al. Prognostic factors identifying biochemical recurrence in patients with positive margins after radical prostatectomy. Int Urol Nephrol. 2011;43(3):715–20.
46. Godoy G, Tareen BU, Lepor H. Site of positive surgical margins influences biochemical recurrence after radical prostatectomy. BJU Int. 2009;104(11):1610–4.
47. Bastide C, Savage C, Cronin A, Zelefsky MJ, Eastham JA, Touijer K, et al. Location and number of positive surgical margins as prognostic factors of biochemical recurrence after salvage radiation therapy after radical prostatectomy. BJU Int. 2010;106(10):1454–7.
48. Salomon L, Anastasiadis AG, Levrel O, Katz R, Saint F, de la Taille A, et al. Location of positive surgical margins after retropubic, perineal, and laparoscopic radical prostatectomy for organ-confined prostate cancer. Urology. 2003;61(2):386–90.
49. Guillonneau B, el-Fettouh H, Baumert H, Cathelineau X, Doublet JD, Fromont G, et al. Laparoscopic radical prostatectomy: oncological evaluation after 1,000 cases a Montsouris Institute. J Urol. 2003;169(4):1261–6.
50. Smith JA, Chan RC, Chang SS, Herrell SD, Clark PE, Baumgartner R, et al. A comparison of the incidence and location of positive surgical margins in robotic assisted laparoscopic radical

prostatectomy and open retropubic radical prostatectomy. J Urol. 2007;178(6):2385–9; discussion 2389–90
51. Patel VR, Coelho RF, Rocco B, Orvieto M, Sivaraman A, Palmer KJ, et al. Positive surgical margins after robotic assisted radical prostatectomy: a multi-institutional study. J Urol. 2011;186(2):511–6.
52. Dev HS, Wiklund P, Patel V, Parashar D, Palmer K, Nyberg T, et al. Surgical margin length and location affect recurrence rates after robotic prostatectomy. Urol Oncol. 2015;33(3):109.e7–13.
53. Barakat B, Othman H, Gauger U, Wolff I, Hadaschik B, Rehme C. Retzius sparing radical prostatectomy versus robot-assisted radical prostatectomy: which technique is more beneficial for prostate cancer patients (MASTER study)? A systematic review and meta-analysis. Eur Urol Focus. 2022;8(4):1060–71.
54. Wagaskar VG, Mittal A, Sobotka S, Ratnani P, Lantz A, Falagario UG, et al. Hood technique for robotic radical prostatectomy-preserving periurethral anatomical structures in the space of Retzius and sparing the pouch of Douglas, enabling early return of continence without compromising surgical margin rates. Eur Urol. 2021;80(2):213–21.
55. Coakley FV, Eberhardt S, Kattan MW, Wei DC, Scardino PT, Hricak H. Urinary continence after radical retropubic prostatectomy: relationship with membranous urethral length on preoperative endorectal magnetic resonance imaging. J Urol. 2002;168(3):1032–5.
56. Ko YH, Huynh LM, See K, Lall C, Skarecky D, Ahlering TE. Impact of surgically maximized versus native membranous urethral length on 30-day and long-term pad-free continence after robot-assisted radical prostatectomy. Prostate Int. 2020;8(2):55–61.
57. Mungovan SF, Sandhu JS, Akin O, Smart NA, Graham PL, Patel MI. Preoperative membranous urethral length measurement and continence recovery following radical prostatectomy: a systematic review and meta-analysis. Eur Urol. 2017;71(3):368–78.
58. Brockman JA, Alanee S, Vickers AJ, Scardino PT, Wood DP, Kibel AS, et al. Nomogram predicting prostate cancer-specific mortality for men with biochemical recurrence after radical prostatectomy. Eur Urol. 2015;67(6):1160–7.
59. Abdollah F, Boorjian S, Cozzarini C, Suardi N, Sun M, Fiorino C, et al. Survival following biochemical recurrence after radical prostatectomy and adjuvant radiotherapy in patients with prostate cancer: the impact of competing causes of mortality and patient stratification. Eur Urol. 2013;64(4):557–64.
60. Bianchi L, Schiavina R, Borghesi M, Bianchi FM, Briganti A, Carini M, et al. Evaluating the predictive accuracy and the clinical benefit of a nomogram aimed to predict survival in node-positive prostate cancer patients: External validation on a multi-institutional database. Int J Urol. 2018;25(6):574–81.
61. Miyoshi Y, Noguchi K, Yanagisawa M, Taguri M, Morita S, Ikeda I, et al. Nomogram for overall survival of Japanese patients with bone-metastatic prostate cancer. BMC Cancer. 2015;15:338.
62. Pruthi RS, Johnstone I, Tu IP, Stamey TA. Prostate-specific antigen doubling times in patients who have failed radical prostatectomy: correlation with histologic characteristics of the primary cancer. Urology. 1997;49(5):737–42.
63. Patel A, Dorey F, Franklin J, deKernion JB. Recurrence patterns after radical retropubic prostatectomy: clinical usefulness of prostate specific antigen doubling times and log slope prostate specific antigen. J Urol. 1997;158(4):1441–5.
64. Ahlering TE, Skarecky DW. Long-term outcome of detectable PSA levels after radical prostatectomy. Prostate Cancer Prostatic Dis. 2005;8(2):163–6.
65. Cary KC, Johnson CS, Cheng L, Koch MO. A critical assessment of post-prostatectomy prostate specific antigen doubling time acceleration--is it stable? J Urol. 2012;187(5):1614–9.
66. Huang E, Tran J, Huynh LM, Skarecky D, Wilson RH, Ahlering T. Prostate-specific antigen doubling time kinetics following radical prostatectomy to guide need for treatment intervention: validation of low-risk recurrences. Cancers (Basel). 2022;14(17):4087.
67. Matsumoto K, Niwa N, Hagiwara M, Kosaka T, Tanaka N, Takeda T, et al. Type of patients in whom biochemical recurrence after radical prostatectomy can be observed without salvage therapy. World J Urol. 2020;38(7):1749–56.

68. Mottet N, van den Bergh RCN, Briers E, Van den Broeck T, Cumberbatch MG, De Santis M, et al. EAU-EANM-ESTRO-ESUR-SIOG guidelines on prostate cancer-2020 update. Part 1: screening, diagnosis, and local treatment with curative intent. Eur Urol. 2021;79(2):243–62.
69. Huang E, Huynh LM, Tran J, Gordon AM, Chandhoke R, Morales B, et al. Active observation of biochemical recurrence without treatment following radical prostatectomy: long-term analysis of outcomes. Cancers (Basel). 2022;14(17):4078.
70. Kasraeian A, Barret E, Chan J, Sanchez-Salas R, Validire P, Cathelineau X, et al. Comparison of the rate, location and size of positive surgical margins after laparoscopic and robot-assisted laparoscopic radical prostatectomy. BJU Int. 2011;108(7):1174–8.
71. Fleshner NE, Evans A, Chadwick K, Lawrentschuk N, Zlotta A. Clinical significance of the positive surgical margin based upon location, grade, and stage. Urol Oncol. 2010;28(2):197–204.
72. Novara G, Ficarra V, Mocellin S, Ahlering TE, Carroll PR, Graefen M, et al. Systematic review and meta-analysis of studies reporting oncologic outcome after robot-assisted radical prostatectomy. Eur Urol. 2012;62(3):382–404.
73. Sooriakumaran P, Haendler L, Nyberg T, Gronberg H, Nilsson A, Carlsson S, et al. Biochemical recurrence after robot-assisted radical prostatectomy in a European single-centre cohort with a minimum follow-up time of 5 years. Eur Urol. 2012;62(5):768–74.
74. Srivastava A, Chopra S, Pham A, Sooriakumaran P, Durand M, Chughtai B, et al. Effect of a risk-stratified grade of nerve-sparing technique on early return of continence after robot-assisted laparoscopic radical prostatectomy. Eur Urol. 2013;63(3):438–44.
75. Vickers AJ, Bianco FJ, Gonen M, Cronin AM, Eastham JA, Schrag D, et al. Effects of pathologic stage on the learning curve for radical prostatectomy: evidence that recurrence in organ-confined cancer is largely related to inadequate surgical technique. Eur Urol. 2008;53(5):960–6.
76. Tewari AK, Srivastava A, Mudaliar K, Tan GY, Grover S, El Douaihy Y, et al. Anatomical retro-apical technique of synchronous (posterior and anterior) urethral transection: a novel approach for ameliorating apical margin positivity during robotic radical prostatectomy. BJU Int. 2010;106(9):1364–73.
77. Sooriakumaran P, Srivastava A, Shariat SF, Stricker PD, Ahlering T, Eden CG, et al. A multinational, multi-institutional study comparing positive surgical margin rates among 22393 open, laparoscopic, and robot-assisted radical prostatectomy patients. Eur Urol. 2014;66(3):450–6.
78. Eastham JA, Kuroiwa K, Ohori M, Serio AM, Gorbonos A, Maru N, et al. Prognostic significance of location of positive margins in radical prostatectomy specimens. Urology. 2007;70(5):965–9.
79. van den Ouden D, Bentvelsen FM, Boevé ER, Schröder FH. Positive margins after radical prostatectomy: correlation with local recurrence and distant progression. Br J Urol. 1993;72(4):489–94.
80. Fesseha T, Sakr W, Grignon D, Banerjee M, Wood DP, Pontes JE. Prognostic implications of a positive apical margin in radical prostatectomy specimens. J Urol. 1997;158(6):2176–9.
81. Patel VR, Thaly R, Shah K. Robotic radical prostatectomy: outcomes of 500 cases. BJU Int. 2007;99(5):1109–12.
82. Ahlering TE, Woo D, Eichel L, Lee DI, Edwards R, Skarecky DW. Robot-assisted versus open radical prostatectomy: a comparison of one surgeon's outcomes. Urology. 2004;63(5):819–22.
83. Tan PH, Cheng L, Srigley JR, Griffiths D, Humphrey PA, van der Kwast TH, et al. International Society of Urological Pathology (ISUP) Consensus Conference on Handling and Staging of Radical Prostatectomy Specimens. Working group 5: surgical margins. Mod Pathol. 2011;24(1):48–57.
84. von Bodman C, Brock M, Roghmann F, Byers A, Löppenberg B, Braun K, et al. Intraoperative frozen section of the prostate decreases positive margin rate while ensuring nerve sparing procedure during radical prostatectomy. J Urol. 2013;190(2):515–20.

8 Challenging Scenarios in Radical Prostatectomy: How to Ensure Similar Functional Outcomes

Shirin Razdan, Sneha Parekh, and Sanjay Razdan

Introduction

In the last two decades, with evolving data on the functional and oncological outcomes of post-robot-assisted laparoscopic prostatectomy (RALP), best practice recommendations have been generated [1]. Since the first RALP performed in 2000, urologists have come across various complex cases of RALP. These complex cases include RALP after a prior transurethral resection of prostate (TURP), cases with large prostate (LP), large median lobe (LML), narrow and deep pelvis, RALP in obese men, RALP after prior renal transplant, prior multiple prostate biopsies, and

Supplementary Information The online version contains supplementary material available at https://doi.org/10.1007/978-3-031-64245-6_8.

S. Razdan
Miami Robotic Surgery at the Comprehensive Urologic Surgery Institute, Miami, FL, USA

S. Parekh
Larkin Palm Springs Hospital, Hialeah, FL, USA

S. Razdan (✉)
International Robotic Institute for Prostate Cancer, Miami, FL, USA

S. Razdan, S. Razdan (eds.), *Urinary Continence and Sexual Function After Robotic Prostatectomy, Radiation, and Novel Therapies*,
https://doi.org/10.1007/978-3-031-64245-6_8

prior suprapubic prostatectomy. In these scenarios similar to any RALP case, restoring the distorted pelvic anatomy, fascial architecture, meticulous dissection of fibrosed periprostatic structures, and adhesion and reconstruction with water-tight anastomosis to achieve better oncological and functional outcomes have been the primary objectives. Keeping these objectives in mind, technical modifications that involve preoperative and intraoperative maneuvers have been developed. These include preoperative multidisciplinary planning [2, 3], detailed information about prior procedure, proximal port placement [4], intraoperative use of dyes for visualizing ureteric orifices [5], use of newer 8-mm cameras [6], changing the 30–70° lens at appropriate steps, fourth-arm use and traction-countertraction maneuver to enhance visualization, and dissection of the anatomical planes in the operative field [7, 8]. Moreover, the learning curve has been found to be a major contributor in the ability of a surgeon to overcome these challenges [9, 10]. With increasing cases and experience, a natural trend to perform more complex cases and implement technical tips and tricks in such challenging cases is noted [11, 12].

Challenging Scenarios

Post-Transurethral Resection of Prostate (TURP) and Its Modifications

Challenges

Any prior procedure on the prostate runs the risk of disruption of normal anatomy, specifically the urethral and bladder neck (BN) anatomy. A TURP risks perforating the prostatic capsule, with extravasation of fluid and blood leading to fibrosis and periprostatic adhesions. This affects neurovascular bundle (NVB) identification and precise surgical dissection that results in worse functional outcomes [13]. The fibrosis caused by the extravasated fluid and removal of tissue in a TURP makes the prostatovesical junction floppy, making its identification difficult. This hinders the preservation of an adequate urethral length and achieving an adequate vesicourethral anastomosis (VUA), which influences functional outcomes. Scarring at the BN further pulls the ureteric orifices closer to the BN and makes visualization of the BN and orifices difficult. The wide BN post-TURP increases the need for a BN reconstruction that may have an impact on anastomotic leakage and continence post-RALP. The cicatrized tissue of BN impairs the healing of the VUA, resulting in prolonged urinary leakage. Moreover, TURP involves the application of thermal energy via monopolar or bipolar cautery on the delicate soft tissue of the urethra and affects the internal and external sphincter mechanisms, making them deficient, and urethral manipulation increases the risk of late stricture formation [14]. TURP generates reactive changes and causes enlargement of the lymph node, which is difficult to interpret on preoperative imaging for preoperative planning. The continuous fluid irrigation in TURP opens the lymphovascular channels and increases the risk of metastasis [15].

Technical Tips and Results

A meta-analysis of 13 studies compared intra- and postoperative outcomes in men undergoing open, laparoscopic, or robotic prostatectomy with prior TURP with men who did not have a prior TURP. Men with prior TURP were shown to have poorer oncological outcomes, higher BN reconstruction rate, and overall higher complication rate post-RALP. No difference was noted in operative time (OT), blood loss, and 1-year urinary continence rate between the two groups [16]. Within the last decade, robotics has drastically changed the outcomes post-RALP [17].

BN Identification and Sparing

Preoperative or intraoperative cystoscopy helps visualize the anatomical distortion of BN, ureteral orifices, and prostate-vesical junction in post-TURP cases [11]. Coelho et al. [18] described the initial step in understanding the anatomy by carefully entering the bladder in the midline, gently grasping the prostate, and examining the prostatic anatomy internally. To keep in mind the positioning of the foley balloon in these prior TURP cases, which might be situated in the prostatic urethra instead of the BN that can mislead the surgeon to overdissect the BN tissue and violate the prostate. To facilitate posterior BN dissection, the fourth robotic arm was used to grasp the posterior prostate, and the posterior BN was grasped with a Maryland bipolar forcep. This helps provide a clear visualization and a sufficient working space. Su et al. [19] used prior resection margin as the demarcation point for achieving a proper plane of BN dissection after initial identification and entry into the BN. Post-TURP BN sparing is seldom performed, but the wide BN in this study was reconstructed following the prior resection plane. The author found that previous surgery has no effect on oncological and functional outcomes, EBL, and OT. Men with prior TURP had weak urine stream at 12 months post-RALP vs non-TURP patients. Tugcu et al. [14] considered RALP following prior intervention as an oncologically promising procedure, but with a longer console time, longer anastomosis time, higher EBL, and higher anastomotic stricture rate.

Endopelvic Fascia Sparing and High Release of Prostatic Fascia

Hampton et al. [20] in 2008 analyzed the positive surgical margin (PSM) rate in men undergoing RALP. The "veil of Aphrodite" technique described by Menon et al. [21] with endopelvic fascia sparing and high release of the prostatic fascia was implemented. The authors found that men with prior TURP have significantly higher PSM than in men who did not have prior TURP (35.3% vs 17.6%). The highest effect of this was at the BN, hence considering frozen section analysis of the BN may reduce the incidence of a positive margin in these cases.

Maximal Urethral Length Preservation (MULP) Technique

Razdan et al. [12] studied the impact of prior TURP on overall difficulty of RALP, biochemical recurrence (BCR)-free rates, and functional outcomes when performed by experienced surgeons with a minimum time interval of 3 months between TURP and RALP. The authors performed the maximum urethral length preservation (MULP) [22] technique for all patients. After entering the BN, posterior dissection, antegrade NS, and dorsal venous complex (DVC) dissection, the prostatic apex and rhabdosphincter are visualized, and apical dissection begins. It starts from the prostatic-rhabdosphincter junction by division of the striated and the smooth muscle fibers traversing from the apex toward the membranous urethra. This is performed with a robotic endo shear along the retroapical plane. The robotic fourth arm was used for twisting and rotating the prostate from side to side for distinct visualization of the apex that helped prevent inadvertent capsulotomy or leaving a PSM. Subsequent dissection of the flimsy posterior prostatic connections at the apex allowed exposure of an additional length of intraprostatic urethra, which is then preserved and added to the MULP. After this careful dissection is complete and the urethra is divided at the new prostate-urethral junction, a long urethral stump is preserved. At the end, van Velthoven technique was used for achieving a water-tight VUA. The authors found no significant difference in potency and continence rates at 1-year and 3-year time interval in both groups ($p = 0.5$). Comparable rates of complications ($p = 0.3$), PSM ($p = 0.4$), extracapsular disease ($p = 0.3$), or seminal vesicle (SV) invasion ($p = 0.1$) were found among both the groups. However, PSM rates were 60% vs 13.5% at BN and 32% vs 31% at the apex in prior TURP group vs TURP naive group, respectively. Hence, the BN is at a higher risk and apex at a lower risk of having a PSM. This finding of higher risk of PSM at BN is in synchrony with the outcomes mentioned in prior literature [23, 24].

Total Anatomical Reconstruction (TAR)

Campobasso et al. [25] in his study of patients with a prior TURP who underwent RALP with TAR demonstrated 95% continence rate at 1 year, PSM present in only 20% cases, with no intraoperative events. These results are comparable with their previous study on patients who underwent RALP with TAR but no prior TURP procedure [26]. The TAR involves a triple-layer posterior reconstruction using a 3–0 barbed suture. The first layer is reconstructed by passing the needle through the cranial portion of previously sectioned Denonvilliers' fascia and the median raphe moving from right to left. The second layer involves suturing the retrotrigonal fascia and the median raphe moving from left to right. The third layer involves suturing the bladder neck (excluding the mucosa of the bladder) and the posterior aspect of the rhabdosphincter again moving from right to left. The VUA is performed by a 3-0 barbed running suture involving the full thickness of the bladder and the urethra, starting at 4 o'clock on the urethra and proceeding clockwise [26]. Gupta et al. [11] in their study found similar results of higher PSM, along with greater blood loss (494 vs 324 mL), need for BN reconstruction (26.7% vs 9.7%), longer OT (189 vs 166 minutes), higher incontinence rates at 6 (14% vs 11.8%) and 12 (25% vs 8%) months follow-up, and higher BCR in men with prior TURP undergoing RALP than the control group of TURP-naïve cases.

The longer OT and higher blood loss in the aforementioned studies are accounted by the longer time taken for BN reconstruction and anastomosis. These studies recommend that RALP post-TURP is a safe and feasible option with no significant complications, provided that it is performed by an experienced and skilled surgeon.

Laser Therapy

Over the last two decades, various laser therapies have been developed and used for prostate resection. These include holmium laser enucleation of the prostate (HoLEP), Greenlight KTP 532-nm wavelength photoselective vaporization system, and Thulium continuous wave laser using the metal Thulium [13].

Abedali et al. [27] in his study came across the following challenges intraoperatively in cases undergoing RALP. The application of laser distorts the BN anatomy and tissue architecture, making demarcation of bladder trigone, ureteral orifices, and vesicoprostatic junction difficult. The authors suggest taking additional time for delineating the bladder anatomy and identifying the ureteral orifices before posterior BN dissection. Using methylene blue or indigo carmine can be helpful tools during this step. Furthermore, HoLEP leaves a very thin tissue at the prostatic apex, subjecting the surgeon to inadvertently enter the anterior prostatic capsule that might damage the anterolateral periprostatic nerves. During apical dissection, the authors recommend to have a distal, anterior dissection arc at the prostatic apex to avoid the potential iatrogenic injury to the prostate. Applying these tips in their following series [28], the authors found similar oncological and perioperative outcomes in the matched cohorts. Their study compared the initial intraoperative and functional outcomes in patients undergoing RALP with previous HoLEP to controls as HoLEP-naïve patients. Though the OT was longer (193.5 vs 164.2 minutes, $P < 0.001$) and delayed continence recovery was seen in the prior HoLEP group (20 vs 6 months, $P = 0.007$), the time to continence recovery was shorter in this large cohort series than in the previous initial outcome series (16 vs 36 weeks). Hence, the authors suggest that a learning curve exists even among experienced surgeons in these cases and better results can be achieved with technical familiarity.

Median Lobes (ML)

Challenges

There is a well-established consensus regarding the median lobe (ML) anatomy and its posing challenges encountered by the surgeon during RALP [5, 8]. A large median lobe (LML) obstructs the laminar flow at the BN and distorts the flow channel at the prostatic-urethral angle, being one of the causes of the obstructive symptoms of the lower urinary tract. The LML makes visualization of the ureteral orifices and dissection of the posterior prostate wall difficult. This difficult posterior dissection can injure the bladder wall. Moreover, a large protruding ML impinges the BN over the ureteral orifice and increases the risks of injury to the ureteral orifices.

Techniques and Results

Considering the abovementioned challenges, technical tips have been provided by various studies in the past that have provided promising functional outcomes, with lower PSM rates as described below.

Early BN Release and ML Identification

Huang et al. [7] found that LMLs do have a positive correlation with increased EBL, OT, and length of stay but do not impact functional outcomes. The authors have applied maneuvers at different steps of the procedure as described in detail. BN was initially identified by lifting the bladder in an anterior and cephalad direction using a fourth robotic arm pro-grasper, while blunt dissection peels off the proximal bladder fibers. Blunt dissection was followed until the funneling longitudinal bladder fibers that form the prostatic urethra were identified. Then, bladder fibers were released posterolaterally until the periprostatic fat that is a landmark for the prostatic artery is identified. The authors realized that the presence of a LML contributes to an early inadvertent cystostomy due to the lateral displacement and anterior attenuation of the BN by the LML. In such scenarios, BN preservation was done via dissecting the BN distal to the cystotomy. This cystotomy repair was incorporated in the VUA that starts proximal to the cystotomy and ends through the urethra. While proceeding with further dissection, to minimize the traction on cystostomy, the anterolateral bladder was released prior to anterior BN dissection. Further, a 180-degree circumferential dissection of the BN via blunt dissection using concurrent spreading with the Maryland dissector and a "breast stroke" maneuver with the scissors was done. This helped in the early identification of the ML before performing a sharp division of the anterior BN. After the anterior BN dissection, the catheter was deflated and pulled back for clear visualization of the posterior BN mucosa, achieving an anatomical BN preservation. With a preserved BN, ureteral orifices were safely located proximal to the BN. Avoiding injury to the ureteral orifices during VUA was assured by taking approximately 1 cm bites of the bladder edge, and in cases with a wider BN, an anterior BN reconstruction is performed. After the posterior BN dissection away from the ML, the anatomic plane between the ML, prostatic base, and posterior BN was better identified with retraction on ML and posterior BN. The anterior and caudal retraction was applied on the ML with the fourth arm pro-grasper, and the anterior and cephalad grasper retraction was on the posterior BN. The major drawback in this was inadvertent cystotomy of the posterior BN in a dissection plane proximal to the anatomic posterior prostate-vesical junction. This inadvertent injury to the posterior BN can be avoided by proper identification of circular fibers of the posterior BN and using the posterior bladder mucosa as a reference point when releasing the countertraction on the posterior BN and adjusting the dissection plane accordingly. Further, it should be kept in mind that the Trendelenburg position accentuates the distance of dissection from the prostate base to apex. This necessitates the dissection to be in the posterior and cephalad directions along the anatomic plane of vesicoprostatic junction instead of coursing along the ML curvature that would lead to incomplete prostate resection.

Patel et al. [29] described tips for achieving smaller BN where the robotic fourth arm pro-grasper is used to elevate the ML, which is then incised transversely at the midpoint and a plane of dissection is developed inferiorly and circumferentially across the lobe. While the fourth arm adjusts the lobe position, the assistant suction arm pushes the bladder inferiorly for a clearer dissection. The proximal bladder wall is identified, and hence, a smaller BN is obtained. Hamidi et al. [30] in his study using this technique showed that LML does have an impact in the early return of continence post-RALP, but no effect on PSM, BCR, perioperative complication, and blood loss.

Carter-Thomason Device

One of the studies used the Carter-Thomason device to elevate the prostate and facilitate a better visualization of the posterior plane of dissection. This device elevates the prostate toward the abdominal wall via a suture tied at the distal pore of the foley catheter. It pulls the prostate and SV away from the posterior plane of dissection, which decreases the technical difficulty in performing the posterior BN and SV dissection. Using this technique, the intra-OT was longer in men with a ML than the control group with no ML (280 minutes vs 349 minutes, $P = 0.0058$). Men with LML had a significantly greater incidence of BN reconstruction (40%) than men without ML (14%), However, no significant difference was found in operative complications and continence at 3 and 6 months among both the groups [31].

Large Median Lobe

Sarle et al. [5] in a case report of a 150 g prostate and a ML larger than the prostate described using the following tips intraoperatively. The author used traction, countertraction, and foley catheter to deliver the ML outside the bladder and facilitate dissection of the posterior bladder wall from the prostate. Intraoperative dyes were used to visualize the ureteral orifices, and careful VUA was performed using reverse tennis racquet that involved reconstruction of the posterior plate first and dealing with both ureteral openings at the same time. The postoperative recovery was uneventful, and the patient at 5 days after catheter removal had good urine control with one pad daily for security due to mild stress incontinence. At 18 months follow-up, the patient was completely continent and had resumed preoperative sexual function. Using similar surgical technique, Jenkin et al. [32] in his retrospective study of 345 consecutive patients undergoing RALP compared outcomes in men having ML to men without a ML in their study cohort. Out of the 29 men with ML in their study cohort, 55% of men with ML required BN reconstruction compared with 4% men without a ML. No significant difference was found in OT, EBL, PSM, final pathological stage, complications, and postoperative urinary outcomes (Video 8.1).

Hood Technique of RALP

Wagaskar et al. used the hood technique to compare oncological outcomes in LML with patients with no ML and found extended OT and increased EBL in the former group [33]. The authors in this study describe the following maneuvers that can help face the challenges in cases with a ML and LML. After developing the retropubic space, the anterior BN is incised until the foley catheter is seen, and then a Foley catheter is grasped by the tip with firm anterior traction. The ML is identified and stay sutures are placed to deliver it outside the BN. The ML is delivered using a 3-0 Vicryl suture, and tenaculum forceps are used instead of ProGrasp forceps in cases of huge MLs (>2.5 cm in size). Delivering the ML out of the BN helps in better visualization of ureteric orifices. This can be confirmed through direct visualization of urine flow from the ureteric orifices or intraoperative use of Lasix, indocyanine green, or methylene blue. This is followed by the identification of the retrotriagonal layer and dissection of SV and vas deferens (VD). The development of this layer can be improved with an assistant holding the ML high via stray sutures on the ML, holding the posterior edge of the prostate, and an assistant holding the posterior bladder wall. With serial traction and countertraction, a plane is developed between the prostate capsule and Denonvilliers' fascia for nerve sparing (NS). This plane of NS is followed distally toward the apex and laterally on the sides. The prostatic pedicles are cut, followed by the anterolateral dissection of the prostate on both sides. Two ports are used by the assistant, one hand is used for the retraction of the prostate and other hand for traction and countertraction for NS. A plane is created anteriorly between the detrusor apron and anterior fibromuscular stroma that leads to the preservation of the anterolateral periprostatic structures, aka hood. The DVC is ligated using 2-0 Vicryl suture in a continuous fashion followed by circumferential apical dissection and meticulous urethral transection. The prostate is removed out of the operative field, and the procedure is completed with total anatomical reconstruction. The posterior BN reconstruction is performed by developing a "mattress" for anastomosis using V-lock suture. A two-layer BN reconstruction is performed, and a water-tight, tension-free VUA is completed using 3-0 Stratafix suture. Patients with a ML had statistically significant higher median prostate-specific antigen (PSA; 7.7 vs 5.8 ng/dl), PSA density (0.17 vs 0.09), and International Prostate Symptom Score (19.5 vs 7.2); longer median console time (114 vs 134 minutes) and surgery time (145 vs 170 minutes); and higher blood loss (150 vs 175 ml) than men without a ML. There were no statistically significant differences found in pathological stages (T2, T3; 87%, 13% vs 88%, 12%) and rates of PSM (7% vs 8.5%) between both groups. The authors suggest that RALP is challenging in cases with a LML and has a steep learning curve. Understanding the key steps to facilitate BN dissection can help avoid intraoperative events and achieve best possible functional outcomes.

Large Prostates (LP)

Challenges

The challenges with LP are the visualization of the periprostatic field, creating precise dissection planes, and blood loss. The thickened bladder wall secondary to bladder outlet obstruction distorts the uniformity of bladder wall thickness, making the vesicourethral anastomosis difficult [11].

Technique and Results

Asynchronous NS

As described above for ML, Huang et al. when using his technique of RALP mentioned NS to be a challenging step due to the limited pelvic space available with the presence of the large gland. The mass effect secondary to the large gland displaces the NVBs posteriorly, making the visualization of the NVB during NS difficult, particularly at the apex that makes NS asynchronous. The authors performed asynchronous NS, a division of detrusor apron and DVC midway after ceasing the antegrade NS at the level of mid-prostate. This enhances the visualization at the apex for further traction-free NS toward the apex. This step avoids the excessive prostate rotation and medial traction that are performed to reach the posterior apex during the circumferential apical dissection [7].

Early Endopelvic Fascia Opening and DVC Ligation

Using the technique of clipless antegrade NVB preservation during RALP, [34] Marchetti and colleagues [35] evaluated the impact of prostate weight (PW) on the probability of having a PSM in patients undergoing RALP for low-risk prostate cancer. The authors use a transperitoneal (TP) approach to enter the pelvic cavity, SVs and VDs are dissected, then the bladder is completely mobilized, and the endopelvic fascia is opened. This was followed by DVC suture ligation and division, BN opening, and NS in an antegrade fashion. The VUA is performed via the van Velthoven running suture technique with Lapra-Ty clips. Technical innovation of incising/opening the endopelvic fascia followed by early DVC ligation helps control vascular supply and hence blood loss. The authors showed that low PW is independently associated with PSM, which is supported by many other previous studies, but no association with functional outcome [36] [37]. Using similar operative technique, Alenizi et al. [38] found that larger prostate volume (PV) has a positive correlation with a longer OT (OR 1.04). Kim et al. [39]

in his single surgeon series of extraperitoneal (EP) RALP, where the endopelvic fascia was also incised first prior to apical and NVB dissection, analyzed the surgical and oncological outcomes in their study cohort. The study demonstrated significant differences in his cohorts with PW < 25 g, 25–50 g, 50–75 g, and >75 g for console time, EBL, extracapsular extension, pathological score, and stage but did not show any significant difference in oncologic outcome and intraoperative complications. This suggests that EP-RALP requires meticulous hemostasis in patients with a prostate weighing >75 g, and if appropriate management is implemented for blood loss intraoperatively, EP-RALP can be performed regardless of the prostate size.

Early Lymphadenectomy, Wide Bladder Descent, and BN Preservation

Contrary to the conventional RALP procedure, where lymphadenectomy is performed after complete prostate excision, Tewari et al. [40] performed bilateral pelvic lymphadenectomy before RP in a case with large prostate as explained here. It can be performed for large prostates that fill the pelvic cavity and extend from one obturator fossa to the other. This helps in avoiding injury to the obturator and iliac vessels and better determines the lateral surgical boundaries. In cases where lymphadenectomy is done post-prostate excision, wide descent of bladder can be adopted to achieve better surgical exposure of the pelvic cavity. Care must be taken not to enter in the adenoma plane and leave behind the peripheral zone of the prostate. After posterior BN dissection, foley catheter traction is applied in the anterior and cephalad direction for facilitating SV and VD dissection. Whenever this maneuver is not sufficient, a 0 or 2-0 absorbable traction suture on a large needle can be applied at the prostate base. These maneuvers help in achieving wider surgical exposure and bloodless surgical field. In this study, to avoid PSM at the prostate base, BN was not preserved and was reconstructed in the anterior "tennis racket" fashion after completing the VUA. The authors found that robotic approach for large prostates gives promising oncological results but needs longer OT and has higher EBL than in cases with smaller glands.

Along with performing these above-described maneuvers, Rajih et al. [41] performed BN preservation whenever feasible based on the preoperative oncological characteristics and intraoperative anatomy. The authors described the preservation of circular bladder neck fibers with tight BN dissection allowing minimal but sufficient visualization of the bladder interior mucosa and ureteral orifices. This study showed that BN preservation (hazard ratio [HR] 0.71; 95% confidence interval [CI] 0.5–0.99; $p = 0.04$) and large PV are predictors of urinary incontinence post-RALP.

Other Results

Acquati et al. [42] in a series of 1831 men who underwent RALP stratified the study cohort into four different groups as prostate weight (PW) of <30 gm, 30 to 49.9 gm, 50 to 69.9 gm, and >70 gm. Patients with prostate >70 gm had higher pretreatment PSA (median 5.8 ng/ml), higher AUA-SS (median 9), longer OT (median 80 minutes), and higher estimated blood loss (EBL) (median 100 cc) ($p < 0.001$ for all variables). Positive surgical margin (PSM) was lower in men with prostate >70 gm compared with other groups with PW < 70 gm (14.4% vs 12.5% vs 10.2% vs 7.2%, respectively, $p < 0.001$). Potency rates were lower at 4 weeks and 3 months in PW > 70 gm and same in all the groups after 6 months, but these potency rates were not statistically significant.

Labanaris et al. [43], in his study, compared outcomes in cases with pathological PW > 100 gms vs controls with prostate size <50 gm. In this study, sexual function was worse at 12 months (61.9% vs 71.2%) with higher OT, EBL, and complications compared with the controls.

Prior Abdominal or Pelvic Surgery (PAPS)

Challenges

Prior abdominal or pelvic surgery leads to adhesions, scarring in the abdominal cavity, and fibrosis in the periprostatic region. These obliterate the anatomical cavities like the space of Retzius around the BN and distort the anatomical planes such as the periprostatic fascial architecture. This disturbs the natural course of the most crucial steps of RALP like VUA and NS, which has an effect on the functional outcomes post-RALP.

Moreover, with robotics the main challenge is gaining access and exposure through the ports and not pelvic dissection in cases with PAPS. The abdominal adhesions make the port insertion for gaining initial access to the cavity difficult, which necessitates adaptation of maneuvers like extensive adhesiolysis and being careful to avoid injuring the surrounding organs [44].

Technique and Results

With the advancements in the da Vinci robotic system, techniques of modified access and pneumoperitoneum development, increased anatomical literature, and the advancing learning curve of surgeons, the earlier reports of prior abdominal/pelvic surgeries leading to a longer OT and higher complication rate in patients undergoing RALP have been contradicted by a series of recent studies [45, 46].

Surgical and oncological outcomes have been previously reported in men undergoing RALP with different prior abdominal surgeries like hernia repair, bilateral ureteral reimplantation, extensive abdominal surgery following multiple gunshot wounds, gastrectomy, and cholecystectomy [3, 47, 48] (Videos 8.2 and 8.3).

Multidisciplinary Approach

The challenges mentioned above can be overcome by preoperative counseling in men undergoing PAPS and categorized under high-risk category for prostate cancer. This can be aided by a multidisciplinary approach involving general surgeons in preoperative planning, which makes them available during the RALP and provides extra set of experienced hands in dealing with the complex anatomy [3]. In a single surgeon series of 2056 RALP cases between March 2003 and July 2011, a total of 420 cases had a PAPS. A multidisciplinary approach was adopted, involving the general surgeon in presurgical planning. The general surgeon was consulted 30% of times, allowing for preserved operative times. Though the OT was increased in cases with the presence of adhesions ($n = 47$) (154 vs 120 minutes, $p < 0.001$), the longest mean OT for a major abdominal surgery was comparable with the mean OT from a meta-analysis of RALP cohorts (154 minutes). This collaborative approach prevented complications and resulted in better surgical outcomes. This study had comparable oncological and functional outcomes among cases with prior surgery and controls with no prior surgery at 1 year follow-up.

Veress Needle vs Hasson vs. Minilaparotomy

For initial access, general surgeons have described using a Veress needle for creating pneumoperitoneum. The insertion of a needle is usually through the abdominal midline at the umbilicus or left upper quadrant, aka Palmer's point [49, 50]. This is the point 3 cm below the left costal margin in the midclavicular line, which is considered the safer area excluding cases with distended abdomen and splenomegaly [51]. A Veress needle is blind and has a risk of causing major vascular injuries. The optic technique of blind trocar insertion or Hasson technique of port insertion are also considered safer than the Veress needle. The Hasson technique has been reported specifically useful for patients with PAPS, midline incisions, and obesity. It involves directly incising the abdominal wall layers, cutting into the peritoneum, and entering the abdomen with a trocar [52]. Here, the surgeons make the first incision lateral to the scar followed by the Hasson technique to insert the trocars that helps overcome the problem of adhesions and enhances visualization. The greater time needed and difficulty in maintaining the pneumoperitoneum limit its use in all patients. A single surgeon series compared outcomes in men with PAPS ($n = 92$) with men without a PAPS ($n = 247$), out of the 392 men in their study who underwent RALP. The author used a similar technique of Hassan access. The study reported similar findings of OT (257 vs 260 minutes), length of stay (7.1 vs 7.2, $p = 0.51$), PSM rate (16.3 vs 12.5%, $p = 0.233$), and complication rate (31.5 vs 26.7%, $p = 0.187$). No significant difference was found in oncological and functional outcomes (continence 100 vs 97%, $p = 0.397$, and potency 62.2 vs 69.5%, $p = 0.460$) at 3 years follow-up [53]. Kashimoto et al. [47] also used the Hasson technique typically performed above the umbilicus, where a six-trocar system placed at least 8 cm apart was their standard practice. Once the pneumoperitoneum was obtained, initial adhesions were cut with laparoscopic scissors through the 8 mm robotic port. Deep pelvic adhesions were removed with robot assistance after the robotic ports had been placed. The authors found no effect of a prior surgery on EBL, PSM rates, mean duration of catheterization, and complication rates. However, the authors found a significant difference in port insertion time among men with prior abdominal surgery and controls without prior abdominal surgery (22 minutes (5–76) vs 17 minutes (7–90), $p = 0.01$). The authors also found that in cases with prior appendectomy that led to peritonitis, additional ports might be required to overcome the complex anatomy, and in cases of inguinal herniorrhaphy that develop mesh plug infection, longer port insertion times may be required.

The adhesions from a prior surgery occasionally require enterolysis prior to complete port placement [44].

A minilaparotomy incision of 4–6 cm for adhesiolysis and fascial closure post-port insertion helps with a clear visualization and safe trocar insertion [54].

The newer da Vinci robotic 8 mm cameras as compared with the conventional 12 mm cameras have helped avoid abdominal trauma, and this miniaturized camera can be inserted through any of the ports, making visualization and access technically more feasible [6].

Prior Inguinal Herniorrhaphy with Mesh

Prior inguinal hernia repair with a mesh has reports of obliterating the space of Retzius and making radical prostatectomy difficult. A case report by Cooperberg and colleagues [45] on RALP in a patient with prior laparoscopic inguinal hernia repair required mesh removal and debridement of anterior abdominal wall, complicating the VUA. While mesh induces scarring in the space of Retzius, a retropubic prostatectomy can still be a feasible option. Technical modifications such as not placing the mesh significantly inferior to the pubic ramus and using two pieces of mesh placed bilaterally but sparing the midline, rather than placing a single large piece across the midline during mesh placement, need to be considered in men more than 50 years of age and more than 40 years with risk factors for prostate cancer present [55, 56]. In a study by Ginzburg et al. [47]. the authors realized the similar difficulty of mesh obliterating the space of Retzius and mesh being densely adherent to the bladder midline. The robotic approach requires going directly through the mesh to access the desired dissection planes. They used Hassan-type access to the peritoneal cavity and port placement under direct vision as necessary. The authors suggest that RALP can safely be performed in cases with prior abdominal surgery and extensive adhesions with no significant effect on overall OT, console time, margin positivity, or incidence of complications in patients undergoing RALP. Additionally, pre-RALP during an inguinal hernia mesh repair, an extraperitoneal herniorrhaphy can facilitate future TP RALPs [48].

Extraperitoneal (EP) vs Transperitoneal (TP)

Considering the following findings from current literature on peritoneal access (extra vs trans vs intra) for individual surgical scenarios can be helpful. Though no differences have been noted in various studies [57], it is believed that extraperitoneal approach has lesser chances of bowel injury and urine leak, making this a better approach for cases with PAPS. However, it is suggested to follow the extraperitoneal approach only after gaining experience in the technique [47]. TP approach can be favored in cases involving extensive lymphadenectomy. Few studies have analyzed the clinical outcomes between the peritoneal approaches (extraperitoneal vs intraperitoneal vs transperitoneal) in men undergoing RALP [57, 58]. No significant difference is noted in surgical and functional outcomes. Horovitz et al. [48] compared EP vs TP approach for initial access to the pelvic cavity and creating the surgical field. The authors in this retrospective study of 2927 RALP cases compared outcomes between 340 EP and 280 TP cases. They found that the TP approach took longer OT, required extensive adhesiolysis, and has longer length of stay post-RALP, slightly lower EBL, and higher overall complications, but these results were not statistically significant.

Narrow and Deep Pelvis

Challenges

The prostate is compactly surrounded by various anatomical structures that play a vital role in continence and sexual function preservation post-RALP. Adequate mobility of the prostate and robotic arms is crucial for delicate maneuvering of the periprostatic structures and achieving better oncological and functional outcomes. However, a complex pelvic anatomy with narrow and deeper pelvis limits the working space, increases the OT and EBL, and affects oncological and functional outcomes [59–61].

Technique and Results

Patient Positioning, Port Placement, and Reconstruction

Several maneuvers have been described in the literature to overcome the difficulties encountered during RALP in men with narrow pelvis. A steep Trendelenburg position can avoid fat and bowel from coming down into the operative field. Increasing the head angle down from the usual 25° to 30° and changing the camera angle from 30° to 0° for later steps of apical dissection and anastomosis can be adapted for better visualization of the operative field. The newer AirSeal® trocar technology commonly used in laparoscopic procedures keeps the intra-abdominal pressure at less than 8 mm Hg and maintains sufficient working space in cases with narrow pelvis. Port placements 0.5 cm higher than the usual position and depressing the instruments can help avoid hitting the pelvic cavity structures and provide easy passage of the instruments toward the operative field. VUA, being one of the most important steps in RALP, is affected in cases with narrow and deep pelvis, due to limited mobility, visibility, and reach of the robotic arms. After prostate removal, surgical reconstruction techniques like using interrupted sutures, two independent running sutures, bidirectional pre-tied running sutures, bidirectional van Velthoven method, unidirectional or bidirectional barbed sutures, and Rocco's stitch for posterior reconstruction increase the urethral stability and decrease the anastomotic tension between the urethra and the BN. These help achieve a water-tight VUA and good continence outcomes [4].

Some maneuvers to avoid clashing of the robotic arms externally like keeping a minimum distance of 8 cm between the arms, depressing the fourth arm, and elevating and medially rotating the third arm can be tried to decrease the initial learning curve [9].

However, there is data suggesting lesser ability of wrist articulation during RALP in deep pelvis cases, irrespective of surgeon learning curve and experience [62]. This study also showed OT to be higher with increased pelvic depth and prostate volume.

Preoperative Imaging and Pelvimetric Parameters

The rising use of imaging pre-RALP has helped guide subsequent surgical dissection. Mason et al. measured various parameters like PV, anteroposterior inlet distance, pelvic depth, anteroposterior distance at midpelvis, pelvic outlet, interspinous distance, intertuberous distance, and pelvic cavity index (PCI). These parameters were statistically analyzed to obtain their correlation with EBL and OT [63]. They found that PV to PCI ratio significantly predicts EBL and OT. Their study also revealed that cases with apical PSM had statistically narrower and deeper pelvis. Hence, meticulous apical dissection is suggested in cases with complex and narrow pelvic anatomy. This subgroup analysis is in accordance with the study results on apical prostate depth (APD) by Matikainen et al. [64], where APD is found to be an independent predictor of apical surgical margin status, independent of surgical approach and pathologic grade and stage. The former multiethnic cohort study found that African-American men have a significantly narrower mid-pelvis, smaller mid-pelvic area, and steeper symphysis pubis angles than their White counterparts. African-American men had a higher impact of having a deep pelvis associated with higher PSM rates [65]. On the contrary, Hong et al. [66] in his study on Korean men did not show any significant association of pelvic dimensions with EBL and OT, which does suggest interindividual and ethnic variations of physical build in pre-RALP planning.

However, Yao et al. [67] suggested that surgeon experience and improved surgical technique can help overcome the technical issues encountered with cases of narrow and deep pelvic anatomy. Out of the many pelvimetry findings, they concluded that PV to PCI was significantly correlated with console time and EBL.

Obese Patient

Challenges

Obesity is a major healthcare problem affecting people in all ages and genders. According to the National Health and Nutrition Examination Survey (NHANES), 42.4% of the US population is obese with body mass index (BMI) > 30. Obesity has been proven to increase the risk of having prostate cancer and has its own genetic basis. The excess abdominal fat makes it more difficult to have access to the pelvic organs if present along with the deeper and narrow pelvis combined with occasional exostosis of the pubic symphysis. The abdominal contour places the ports at an acute angulation and makes it difficult for the ports to easily articulate the robotic arms into the depth of the pelvis. Additionally, the narrow and deep pelvis along with the excess abdominal and periprostatic fat pushes the bladder deeper into the pelvic cavity, obscuring the working space and visual field. A clear field of visualization is important for precise periprostatic fascial dissection and approximating the retractile urethra with the BN for a leak-free VUA [4].

Tips

Certain tips and tricks similar to the ones mentioned for men with narrow pelvis have also been implemented for obese patients. The acute angulations secondary to protuberant abdominal curvature can be overcome by proximal port placement at a distance of approximately 15–18 cm from pubic symphysis. In obese patients with large prostates, BN plication can be performed. Changing the 30-degree lens to 0 degree and depressing the camera port can help overcome the vertical angulation of the ports and avoid hitting the pelvic brim and symphysis pubis. In obese patients, trocars need to be placed deeper into the abdominal cavity, and the robotic arms are deflected laterally to flatten the working angle of the robotic arms for easier reach of the arms into the deeper pelvis. Using bariatric camera and ports can be helpful to traverse the longer axial distance through the abdominal wall. A 12 mm bariatric assistant port pointing toward the umbilicus avoids the port being buried under the preperitoneal fat and potential bowel injury [6].

Results

Results from a national inpatient sample study show that obesity does predispose to higher rates of adverse events at radical prostatectomy (RP) [68]. Body mass index (BMI) has long been proven to be an independent predictive factor for PSM at the apex [69], and Kheterpal et al. [70] in his retrospective study showed men with metabolic syndrome to have worse Gleason grade and pathological stage. Porcaro et al. [71] in his cohort of extended pelvic lymph node dissection found BMI to be an independent predictor of Clavien-Dindo grade 3 complications, increased by 18.4% for each unit rise.

Wiltz et al. recommend that surgeons in their early learning curve phase should be cautious and plan for these technical challenges with cases having BMI >30. The authors demonstrated lower sexual and continence outcomes at 12 and 24 months in obese men and higher EBL and OT. Additionally, increased rates of perioperative complications including aborting cases due to respiratory compromise were noted in more obese men [10]. Xu et al. [72] and Gobler et al. [73] corroborated the aforementioned findings of increased OT and EBL. The authors recommend that the surgeon should wait to perform RALP in obese men until the surgeon overcomes the learning curve. In contrast, a propensity matched score analysis demonstrated no significant difference in OT with higher mean EBL of 113 [41] vs 130 [27] mL in obese men. The surgeons found anastomosis as a difficult step in these men, but the study did not show any statistically significant difference in postoperative complication rates, pain scores, length of stay, and indwelling catheter duration [74]. This is supported by the findings of the study including patient-based model to estimate OTs by Huben et al. [75], where the surgeon was the most strongly associated variable with OT. To reduce risk of perioperative complications, Wilson et al. [76] recommended a low-calorie diet and weight loss program prior to RALP.

Previous Multiple Prostate Biopsies

Challenges

Prostate biopsy leads to tissue inflammation post-biopsy, and in the healing of these inflamed tissues, the cytokines released generate a fibrotic reaction leaving a denser tissue around the prostate. This adherent tissue makes the posterior dissection toward Denonvilliers' fascia and on the posterolateral aspect NS difficult. Repeat biopsies in certain cases of high-grade Gleason (3 + 4 or 4 + 3) on active surveillance (AS) disrupt the neural architecture and periprostatic tissues [77–79].

Tips and Results

Urologists generally follow the protocol of undertaking the patient for a RALP 4–6 weeks post-biopsy for the prostatitis and inflamed tissues to heal [80]. Men at particular risk of post-biopsy inflammatory reaction are those with low-risk disease on AS protocols, as they are subject to repeated biopsies. The repeat biopsies in these men ultimately affect potency and continence function post-RALP [77–79].

Carniero et al. [81] in his prospectively maintained database studied the impact of TRUS biopsies and multiple biopsies on perioperative outcomes like EBL, OT, perioperative complications according to the modified Clavien system, and length of hospital stay. PSM was considered for the oncological outcomes. They found that a higher number of biopsies are related to higher number of complications, and the authors recommended to minimize potential risks of surgical complications in patients who may benefit from RALP. Hence, limiting the number of repeat biopsies in men with clinically significant cancer or using risk-predictive algorithms to avoid unnecessary biopsies can help avoid these complications [82].

Sooriakumaran et al. [83] demonstrated similar results of perioperative complications post-multiple biopsies in men undergoing RALP. In this study, men with prior multiple biopsies had worse erectile function at 3 and 6 months compared with men with prior single biopsy (57% versus 80%). Continence outcomes were not significantly different among both the groups. The authors recommended counseling patients about the risk of impotence who undergo multiple biopsies or opt AS for initial management and later end up with a RALP.

A large population-based cohort study from Ontario demonstrated that men with more than two biopsies had higher perioperative blood transfusion, required more post-RP urodynamic evaluation and BN contracture-related interventions, but were not at increased odds of surgery for incontinence or erectile dysfunction. This study also found that these results can serve as a guide about the risks and safety of multiple prostate biopsies while counseling men on AS [84].

Renal Transplant Recipients

Challenges

The extraperitoneal adhesions from the prior transplant surgery obscure and obliterate the ipsilateral graft site in the retropubic space. The resulted scarring combined with the decreased working space occupied by the renal graft present a unique challenge to the surgeon because of increased adhesions and distorted anatomy.

Tips

Various surgical modifications have been documented for a successful RALP procedure in cases with prior renal transplants. Preoperative assessment of a patient's unique anatomy by revieweing transplant operative notes and surgeon preparedness to convert to an open Hasson technique if Veress access is unsuccessful will allow for successful RALP. Placing and adjusting the ports medial and caudal on the ipsilateral graft site help improve orientation into the pelvis. Meticulous dissection on the posterior prostate needs to be kept in mind due to inadvertent angulations of the port. Using the 30 degree up lens to facilitate dissecting the rectum from the prostate and using the 30 degree down lens instead of 0° for other steps are few of the adaptations a surgeon can take to facilitate RALP after renal transplant. Constant surveillance of the graft and its ureteric anastomosis is of utmost importance at every step [85]. Tewari et al. [86] through a single case report suggested the placement of a bariatric port superolateral to the standard port sites, placing the left port inferolateral to provide adequate access for pelvic lymph node dissection, and developing the retropubic space largely from the contralateral side to avoid allograft injury. The use of perineal approach has been documented to reduce intraoperative iatrogenic injury to the graft, as this approach would avoid the transplant field but lymph node dissection would need a separate incision [85].

Results

A large multicenter study suggested that RALP, though technically challenging, is a feasible technique for treating localized prostate cancer in cases with renal transplants [87]. Leonard et al. in his short series of 27 patients with renal transplants undergoing RALP predicted that renal graft history is an independent risk factor for a shorter BCR-free survival (hazard ratio = 4.291). However, the men in both groups had similar functional, oncological, and complication rates. Moreover, RALP in their series provided a suitable control of the primary tumor, no more morbidity compared with control patients, and acceptable operative risks [88]. Large RCTs can help find the correlation between renal graft history and BCR. Supporting these findings, a French multicenter study also added that RALP does not have any negative impact on the graft renal function and cancer prognosis. Hence, RALP is a conceivable procedure to treat localized prostate cancer in men with a history of renal transplant [89].

After Prior Suprapubic Prostatectomy

Though the number of simple prostatectomies including open and minimally invasive is at a downward trend, open simple prostatectomy is still performed in over >2000 men annually in United States [90]. This accounts for 5% of the total men undergoing prostatectomy in the country; hence, there is still a chance of 1 in 5000 men to undergo RALP after a prior simple prostatectomy [91, 92].

In such scenarios, surgeons encounter intraoperative challenges of complex anatomy, extensive adhesions, distorted anatomical planes, and difficult prostatic dissection and NS. The use of blunt and athermal dissection and a well-experienced surgeon with a large-volume practice can handle these complex atypical anatomical cases better and provide an effective oncological and functional outcome [91, 92].

Razdan et al. [92] described a challenging case of a healthy 61-year-old Hispanic patient, having Gleason 4 + 4 = 8 adenocarcinoma of prostate involving 50–90% of 3 of 12 cores and Gleason 4 + 3 = 7 adenocarcinoma involving 20–85% of 4 of 12 cores on TRUS biopsy. Prostate enlargement was noted on cystoscopy with a scar at the dome of the bladder suggesting prior transvesical approach of prostatectomy.

The authors used a TP four-arm approach of entering the abdomen with a 0-degree lens. After careful colonic mobilization, the anterior bladder was dissected with extensive adhesiolysis from prior surgery. The endopelvic fascia was opened, the BN transected, and the prostate was mobilized. PK scissors were used to perform the blunt posterior dissection to avoid injuring the rectum. Bilateral NS was performed with athermal dissection. Further, BN and apical dissection were done with great caution due to the distorted dissection planes present at these areas from the previous surgery. The MULP technique [22] was used to augment the urethral stump length and achieve MUL possible. The authors tried to achieve a balance between no PSM and achieving best continence outcomes. This patient was completely continent at 2 weeks and was able to maintain erections at 1 month post-RALP with a SHIM score of 22. PSA at 3-month follow-up was <0.1. The authors found that judicious use of thermal energy and blunt dissection at junctures of distorted and challenging anatomy are needed. The author's high volume case experience of RALP (>5000) helped mitigate these intraoperative challenges. Hence, they concluded that RALP is a feasible and safe option in men who have previously undergone suprapubic open prostatectomy for BPH, especially in the hands of an experienced surgeon [92].

Tsui et al. [93] described his experience with a patient who had undergone previous open suprapubic simple prostatectomy. Gentle dissection of bladder from the anterior abdominal wall helped encounter the extensive adhesions. He used the Samadi Modified Advanced Robotic Technique (SMART) to maximize NS, where he did not incise the endopelvic fascia. After opening the BN, ureteral stents were used to identify the exact location of the ureteric orifices. Tissue recognition was challenging at the posterior BN. Athermal technique of NS by blunt dissection with round-tip scissors was implemented. DVC was cut with cold scissors right before the removal of the prostate from the surgical field and later ligated with sutures. The BN was reconstructed in a posterior tennis-racquet fashion with a narrower diameter of 18 Fr., followed by careful bilateral lymph node dissection. Patients at 9 weeks follow-up was found to be continent with no difficulties in voiding and PSA <0.01.

Conclusion

Surgical outcomes post-RALP in challenging cases have been variable and differ mainly based on the surgical experience. This is achieved after overcoming the learning curve. With judicious selection of initial cases in practice and under the presence of an experienced surgeon, the surgical proficiency and dexterity to perform complex cases are achieved. Hence, surgeons can apply the necessary technical modifications described above and achieve desired functional and oncological outcomes.

Take-Home Message

We strove to review some of the more common challenging clinical scenarios that may be encountered by the urologic surgeon. Redo and salvage prostatectomies, patient anatomic limitations, and prior abdominal and pelvic surgeries all contribute to the difficulty of radical prostatectomy. There are both technical nuances and novel technologies and approaches now available that can be employed to overcome these limitations. More recently, the da Vinci Single Port (SP) platform has allowed for an increased ability to perform extraperitoneal and intravesical prostatectomies in men with otherwise hostile abdomens. We advise the junior urologist to carefully note a patient's prior medical and surgical history and meticulously study preoperative prostate MRI to fully understand the challenges that may be encountered at the time of surgery and adequately prepare for them.

References

1. Montorsi F, Wilson TG, Rosen RC, Ahlering TE, Artibani W, Carroll PR, et al. Best practices in robot-assisted radical prostatectomy: recommendations of the Pasadena Consensus Panel. Eur Urol. 2012;62(3):368–81.
2. Burton E, Chase D, Yamamoto M, de Guzman J, Imagawa D, Berman ML. Surgical management of recurrent ovarian cancer: the advantage of collaborative surgical management and a multidisciplinary approach. Gynecol Oncol. 2011;120(1):29–32.
3. Bernstein AN, Lavery HJ, Hobbs AR, Chin E, Samadi DB. Robot-assisted laparoscopic prostatectomy and previous surgical history: a multidisciplinary approach. J Robot Surg. 2013;7(2):143–51.
4. Lu C-H, Ou Y-C. Large volume gland with small pelvis. In: Ren S, Nathan S, Pavan N, Gu D, Sridhar A, Autorino R, editors. Robot-assisted radical prostatectomy: advanced surgical techniques. Cham: Springer International Publishing; 2022. p. 329–34.
5. Sarle R, Tewari A, Hemal AK, Menon M. Robotic-assisted anatomic radical prostatectomy: technical difficulties due to a large median lobe. Urol Int. 2005;74(1):92–4.
6. Darwiche F, Swain S, Kallingal G, Punnen S, Manoharan M, Parekh DJ, et al. Operative technique and early experience for robotic-assisted laparoscopic nephroureterectomy (RALNU) using da Vinci Xi. Springerplus. 2015;4:298.
7. Huang AC, Kowalczyk KJ, Hevelone ND, Lipsitz SR, Yu HY, Plaster BA, et al. The impact of prostate size, median lobe, and prior benign prostatic hyperplasia intervention on robot-assisted laparoscopic prostatectomy: technique and outcomes. Eur Urol. 2011;59(4):595–603.
8. Wagaskar VG, Zaytoun O, Kale P, Pedraza A, Busby D, Reddy A, et al. Technical tips in managing Large median lobes during robot-assisted radical prostatectomy. Eur Urol Open Sci. 2022;45:32–7.
9. Samavedi S, Abdul-Muhsin H, Pigilam S, Sivaraman A, Patel VR. Handling difficult anastomosis. Tips and tricks in obese patients and narrow pelvis. Indian. J Urol. 2014;30(4):418–22.
10. Wiltz AL, Shikanov S, Eggener SE, Katz MH, Thong AE, Steinberg GD, et al. Robotic radical prostatectomy in overweight and obese patients: oncological and validated-functional outcomes. Urology. 2009;73(2):316–22.
11. Gupta NP, Singh P, Nayyar R. Outcomes of robot-assisted radical prostatectomy in men with previous transurethral resection of prostate. BJU Int. 2011;108(9):1501–5.
12. Bajpai RR, Razdan S, Sanchez-Gonzalez MA, Reddy BN. Robot-assisted radical prostatectomy after prior transurethral resection of prostate: an analysis of perioperative, functional, pathologic, and oncologic outcomes. J Endourol. 2022;36(8):1063–9.
13. Lokeshwar SD, Harper BT, Webb E, Jordan A, Dykes TA, Neal DE, et al. Epidemiology and treatment modalities for the management of benign prostatic hyperplasia. Transl Androl Urol. 2019;8(5):529–39.
14. Tugcu V, Atar A, Sahin S, Kargi T, Gokhan Seker K, IlkerComez Y, et al. Robot-assisted radical prostatectomy after previous prostate surgery. JSLS. 2015;19(4):e2015.00080.
15. Acar O, Esen T. Robotic radical prostatectomy in patients with previous prostate surgery and radiotherapy. Prostate Cancer. 2014;2014:367675.
16. Liao H, Duan X, Du Y, Mou X, Hu T, Cai T, et al. Radical prostatectomy after previous transurethral resection of the prostate: oncological, surgical and functional outcomes-a meta-analysis. World J Urol. 2020;38(8):1919–32.
17. Muaddi H, Hafid ME, Choi WJ, Lillie E, de Mestral C, Nathens A, et al. Clinical outcomes of robotic surgery compared to conventional surgical approaches (laparoscopic or open): a systematic overview of reviews. Ann Surg. 2021;273(3):467–73.
18. Rodrigues GJ, Sutherland P, Patel V, Coelho RF. Management of challenging cases during robot-assisted laparoscopic prostatectomy. In: Wiklund P, Mottrie A, Gundeti MS, Patel V, editors. Robotic urologic surgery. Cham: Springer International Publishing; 2022. p. 251–66.

19. Su YK, Katz BF, Sehgal SS, Yu SJ, Su YC, Lightfoot A, et al. Does previous transurethral prostate surgery affect oncologic and continence outcomes after RARP? J Robot Surg. 2015;9(4):291–7.
20. Mandhani A. Prostatic fascia and recovery of sexual function after radical prostatectomy: is it a "Veil of Aphrodite" or "Veil of mystery"! Indian J Urol. 2009;25(1):146–8.
21. Kaul S, Savera A, Badani K, Fumo M, Bhandari A, Menon M. Functional outcomes and oncological efficacy of Vattikuti Institute prostatectomy with Veil of Aphrodite nerve-sparing: an analysis of 154 consecutive patients. BJU Int. 2006;97(3):467–72.
22. Hamada A, Razdan S, Etafy MH, Fagin R. Early return of continence in patients undergoing robot-assisted laparoscopic prostatectomy using modified maximal urethral length preservation technique. J Endourol. 2014;28(8):930–8.
23. Shelfo SW, Obek C, Soloway MS. Update on bladder neck preservation during radical retropubic prostatectomy: impact on pathologic outcome, anastomotic strictures, and continence. Urology. 1998;51(1):73–8.
24. Gacci M, Simonato A, Lanciotti M, Ennas M, Varca V, Maffezzini M, et al. The impact of prior TURP on radical prostatectomy surgical margins: a multicenter analysis. Urol Int. 2013;91(1):62–8.
25. Campobasso D, Fiori C, Amparore D, Checcucci E, Garrou D, Manfredi M, et al. Total anatomical reconstruction during robot-assisted radical prostatectomy in patients with previous prostate surgery. Minerva Urol Nefrol. 2019;71(6):605–11.
26. Porpiglia F, Bertolo R, Manfredi M, De Luca S, Checcucci E, Morra I, et al. Total anatomical reconstruction during robot-assisted radical prostatectomy: implications on early recovery of urinary continence. Eur Urol. 2016;69(3):485–95.
27. Gellhaus PT, Monn MF, Leese J, Flack CK, Lingeman JE, Koch MO, et al. Robot-assisted radical prostatectomy in patients with a history of holmium laser enucleation of the prostate: feasibility and evaluation of initial outcomes. J Endourol. 2015;29(7):764–9.
28. Abedali ZA, Calaway AC, Large T, Koch MO, Lingeman JE, Boris RS. Robot-assisted radical prostatectomy in patients with a history of holmium laser enucleation of the prostate: the Indiana University experience. J Endourol. 2020;34(2):163–8.
29. Patel SR, Kaplon DM, Jarrard D. A technique for the management of a large median lobe in robot-assisted laparoscopic radical prostatectomy. J Endourol. 2010;24(12):1899–901.
30. Hamidi N, Atmaca AF, Canda AE, Keske M, Gok B, Koc E, et al. Does presence of a median lobe affect perioperative complications, oncological outcomes and urinary continence following robotic-assisted radical prostatectomy? Urol J. 2018;15(5):248–55.
31. Meeks JJ, Zhao L, Greco KA, Macejko A, Nadler RB. Impact of prostate median lobe anatomy on robotic-assisted laparoscopic prostatectomy. Urology. 2009;73(2):323–7.
32. Jenkins LC, Nogueira M, Wilding GE, Tan W, Kim HL, Mohler JL, et al. Median lobe in robot-assisted radical prostatectomy: evaluation and management. Urology. 2008;71(5):810–3.
33. Wagaskar VG, Mittal A, Sobotka S, Ratnani P, Lantz A, Falagario UG, et al. Hood technique for robotic radical prostatectomy-preserving periurethral anatomical structures in the space of Retzius and sparing the pouch of Douglas, enabling early return of continence without compromising surgical margin rates. Eur Urol. 2021;80(2):213–21.
34. Chien GW, Mikhail AA, Orvieto MA, Zagaja GP, Sokoloff MH, Brendler CB, et al. Modified clipless antegrade nerve preservation in robotic-assisted laparoscopic radical prostatectomy with validated sexual function evaluation. Urology. 2005;66(2):419–23.
35. Marchetti PE, Shikanov S, Razmaria AA, Zagaja GP, Shalhav AL. Impact of prostate weight on probability of positive surgical margins in patients with low-risk prostate cancer after robotic-assisted laparoscopic radical prostatectomy. Urology. 2011;77(3):677–81.
36. Freedland SJ, Isaacs WB, Platz EA, Terris MK, Aronson WJ, Amling CL, et al. Prostate size and risk of high-grade, advanced prostate cancer and biochemical progression after radical prostatectomy: a search database study. J Clin Oncol. 2005;23(30):7546–54.
37. Pettus JA, Masterson T, Sokol A, Cronin AM, Savage C, Sandhu JS, et al. Prostate size is associated with surgical difficulty but not functional outcome at 1 year after radical prostatectomy. J Urol. 2009;182(3):949–55.

38. Alenizi AM, Valdivieso R, Rajih E, Meskawi M, Toarta C, Bienz M, et al. Factors predicting prolonged operative time for individual surgical steps of robot-assisted radical prostatectomy (RARP): a single surgeon's experience. Can Urol Assoc J. 2015;9(7–8):E417–22.
39. Kim MS, Jang WS, Chung DY, Koh DH, Lee JS, Goh HJ, et al. Effect of prostate gland weight on the surgical and oncological outcomes of extraperitoneal robot-assisted radical prostatectomy. BMC Urol. 2019;19(1):1.
40. El-Hakim A, Leung RA, Richstone L, Kim TS, Te AE, Tewari AK. Athermal robotic technique of prostatectomy in patients with large prostate glands (>75 g): technique and initial results. BJU Int. 2006;98(1):47–9.
41. Rajih E, Meskawi M, Alenizi AM, Zorn KC, Alnazari M, Zanaty M, et al. Perioperative predictors for post-prostatectomy urinary incontinence in prostate cancer patients following robotic-assisted radical prostatectomy: long-term results of a Canadian prospective cohort. Can Urol Assoc J. 2019;13(5):E125–E31.
42. Acquati P, Rocco B, Albo G, Sivaraman A, Chauhan S, Palmer KJ, et al. Does prostate weight affect perioperative outcomes, positive surgical margin rates and functional outcomes after robot-assisted radical prostatectomy performed by an experienced surgeon? 2011.
43. Labanaris AP, Zugor V, Witt JH. Robot-assisted radical prostatectomy in patients with a pathologic prostate specimen weight ≥100 grams versus ≤50 grams: surgical, oncologic and short-term functional outcomes. Urol Int. 2013;90(1):24–30.
44. Ginzburg S, Hu F, Staff I, Tortora J, Champagne A, Salner A, et al. Does prior abdominal surgery influence outcomes or complications of robotic-assisted laparoscopic radical prostatectomy? Urology. 2010;76(5):1125–9.
45. Cooperberg MR, Downs TM, Carroll PR. Radical retropubic prostatectomy frustrated by prior laparoscopic mesh herniorrhaphy. Surgery 2004;135(4):452–3; discussion 4.
46. Berryhill R, Jhaveri J, Yadav R, Leung R, Rao S, El-Hakim A, et al. Robotic prostatectomy: a review of outcomes compared with laparoscopic and open approaches. Urology. 2008;72(1):15–23.
47. Kishimoto N, Takao T, Yamamichi G, Okusa T, Taniguchi A, Tsutahara K, et al. Impact of prior abdominal surgery on the outcomes after robotic – assisted laparoscopic radical prostatectomy: single center experience. Int Braz J Urol. 2016;42(5):918–24.
48. Horovitz D, Feng C, Messing EM, Joseph JV. Extraperitoneal vs. transperitoneal robot-assisted radical prostatectomy in patients with a history of prior inguinal hernia repair with mesh. J Robot Surg. 2017;11(4):447–54.
49. Mayol J, Garcia-Aguilar J, Ortiz-Oshiro E, De-Diego Carmona JA, Fernandez-Represa JA. Risks of the minimal access approach for laparoscopic surgery: multivariate analysis of morbidity related to umbilical trocar insertion. World J Surg. 1997;21(5):529–33.
50. Palmer R. Safety in laparoscopy. J Reprod Med. 1974;13(1):1–5.
51. Ito M, Asano Y, Horiguchi A, Shimizu T, Yamamoto T, Uyama I, et al. Cholecystectomy using single-incision laparoscopic surgery with a new SILS port. J Hepatobiliary Pancreat Sci. 2010;17(5):688–91.
52. Kovachev S, Ganovska A, Atanasova V, Sergeev S, Mutafchiyski V, Vladov N. [Open laparoscopy--a modified Hasson technique]. Akush Ginekol (Sofiia) 2015;54(4):52–56.
53. Di Pierro GB, Grande P, Mordasini L, Danuser H, Mattei A. Robot-assisted radical prostatectomy in the setting of previous abdominal surgery: perioperative results, oncological and functional outcomes, and complications in a single surgeon's series. Int J Surg. 2016;36(Pt A):170–6.
54. Coughlin G, Patel VR. Robot-assisted laparoscopic radical prostatectomy: management of the difficult case. In: Su L-M, editor. Atlas of robotic urologic surgery. Totowa: Humana Press; 2011. p. 79–89.
55. Erdogru T, Teber D, Frede T, Marrero R, Hammady A, Rassweiler J. The effect of previous transperitoneal laparoscopic inguinal herniorrhaphy on transperitoneal laparoscopic radical prostatectomy. J Urol. 2005;173(3):769–72.
56. Lallas CD, Pe ML, Patel JV, Sharma P, Gomella LG, Trabulsi EJ. Transperitoneal robotic-assisted laparoscopic prostatectomy after prosthetic mesh herniorrhaphy. JSLS. 2009;13(2):142–7.

57. Capello SA, Boczko J, Patel HR, Joseph JV. Randomized comparison of extraperitoneal and transperitoneal access for robot-assisted radical prostatectomy. J Endourol. 2007;21(10):1199–202.
58. Madi R, Daignault S, Wood DP. Extraperitoneal v intraperitoneal robotic prostatectomy: analysis of operative outcomes. J Endourol. 2007;21(12):1553–7.
59. Levinson AW, Ward NT, Sulman A, Mettee LZ, Link RE, Su LM, et al. The impact of prostate size on perioperative outcomes in a large laparoscopic radical prostatectomy series. J Endourol. 2009;23(1):147–52.
60. Hsu EI, Hong EK, Lepor H. Influence of body weight and prostate volume on intraoperative, perioperative, and postoperative outcomes after radical retropubic prostatectomy. Urology. 2003;61(3):601–6.
61. Link BA, Nelson R, Josephson DY, Yoshida JS, Crocitto LE, Kawachi MH, et al. The impact of prostate gland weight in robot assisted laparoscopic radical prostatectomy. J Urol. 2008;180(3):928–32.
62. Chen J, Chu T, Ghodoussipour S, Bowman S, Patel H, King K, et al. Effect of surgeon experience and bony pelvic dimensions on surgical performance and patient outcomes in robot-assisted radical prostatectomy. BJU Int. 2019;124(5):828–35.
63. Mason BM, Hakimi AA, Faleck D, Chernyak V, Rozenblitt A, Ghavamian R. The role of preoperative endo-rectal coil magnetic resonance imaging in predicting surgical difficulty for robotic prostatectomy. Urology. 2010;76(5):1130–5.
64. Matikainen MP, von Bodman CJ, Secin FP, Yunis LH, Vora K, Guillonneau B, et al. The depth of the prostatic apex is an independent predictor of positive apical margins at radical prostatectomy. BJU Int. 2010;106(5):622–6.
65. von Bodman C, Matikainen MP, Yunis LH, Laudone V, Scardino PT, Akin O, et al. Ethnic variation in pelvimetric measures and its impact on positive surgical margins at radical prostatectomy. Urology. 2010;76(5):1092–6.
66. Hong SK, Lee ST, Kim SS, Min KE, Hwang IS, Kim M, et al. Effect of bony pelvic dimensions measured by preoperative magnetic resonance imaging on performing robot-assisted laparoscopic prostatectomy. BJU Int. 2009;104(5):664–8.
67. Yao A, Iwamoto H, Masago T, Morizane S, Honda M, Sejima T, et al. Anatomical dimensions using preoperative magnetic resonance imaging: impact on the learning curve of robot-assisted laparoscopic prostatectomy. Int J Urol. 2015;22(1):74–9.
68. Knipper S, Mazzone E, Mistretta FA, Palumbo C, Tian Z, Briganti A, et al. Impact of obesity on perioperative outcomes at robotic-assisted and open radical prostatectomy: results from the National Inpatient Sample. Urology. 2019;133:135–44.
69. Coelho RF, Chauhan S, Orvieto MA, Palmer KJ, Rocco B, Patel VR. Predictive factors for positive surgical margins and their locations after robot-assisted laparoscopic radical prostatectomy. Eur Urol. 2010;57(6):1022–9.
70. Kheterpal E, Sammon JD, Diaz M, Bhandari A, Trinh QD, Pokala N, et al. Effect of metabolic syndrome on pathologic features of prostate cancer. Urol Oncol. 2013;31(7):1054–9.
71. Porcaro AB, Sebben M, Tafuri A, de Luyk N, Corsi P, Processali T, et al. Body mass index is an independent predictor of Clavien-Dindo grade 3 complications in patients undergoing robot assisted radical prostatectomy with extensive pelvic lymph node dissection. J Robot Surg. 2019;13(1):83–9.
72. Xu T, Wang X, Xia L, Zhang X, Qin L, Zhong S, et al. Robot-assisted prostatectomy in obese patients: how influential is obesity on operative outcomes? J Endourol. 2015;29(2):198–208.
73. Goßler C, May M, Rosenhammer B, Breyer J, Stojanoski G, Weikert S, et al. Obesity leads to a higher rate of positive surgical margins in the context of robot-assisted radical prostatectomy. Results of a prospective multicenter study. Cent European. J Urol. 2020;73(4):457–65.
74. Abdul-Muhsin H, Giedelman C, Samavedi S, Schatloff O, Coelho R, Rocco B, et al. Perioperative and early oncological outcomes after robot-assisted radical prostatectomy (RARP) in morbidly obese patients: a propensity score-matched study. BJU Int. 2014;113(1):84–91.

75. Huben NB, Hussein AA, May PR, Whittum M, Krasowski C, Ahmed YE, et al. Development of a patient-based model for estimating operative times for robot-assisted radical prostatectomy. J Endourol. 2018;32(8):730–6.
76. Wilson RL, Shannon T, Calton E, Galvão DA, Taaffe DR, Hart NH, et al. Efficacy of a weight loss program prior to robot assisted radical prostatectomy in overweight and obese men with prostate cancer. Surg Oncol. 2020;35:182–8.
77. Bokhorst LP, Lepistö I, Kakehi Y, Bangma CH, Pickles T, Valdagni R, et al. Complications after prostate biopsies in men on active surveillance and its effects on receiving further biopsies in the Prostate cancer Research International: Active Surveillance (PRIAS) study. BJU Int. 2016;118(3):366–71.
78. Fujita K, Landis P, McNeil BK, Pavlovich CP. Serial prostate biopsies are associated with an increased risk of erectile dysfunction in men with prostate cancer on active surveillance. J Urol. 2009;182(6):2664–9.
79. Zisman A, Leibovici D, Kleinmann J, Siegel YI, Lindner A. The impact of prostate biopsy on patient well-being: a prospective study of pain, anxiety and erectile dysfunction. J Urol. 2001;165(2):445–54.
80. Li J, Jiang Q, Li Q, Zhang Y, Gao L. Does time interval between prostate biopsy and surgery affect outcomes of radical prostatectomy? A systematic review and meta-analysis. Int Urol Nephrol. 2020;52(4):619–31.
81. Carneiro A, Sivaraman A, Sanchez-Salas R, Nunes-Silva I, Baghdadi M, Srougi V, et al. Higher number of transrectal ultrasound guided prostate biopsy cores is associated with higher blood loss and perioperative complications in robot assisted radical prostatectomy. Actas Urol Esp. 2017;41(3):155–61.
82. Parekh S, Ratnani P, Falagario U, Lundon D, Kewlani D, Nasri J, et al. The Mount Sinai prebiopsy risk calculator for predicting any prostate cancer and clinically significant prostate cancer: development of a risk predictive tool and validation with advanced neural networking, prostate magnetic resonance imaging outcome database, and European randomized study of screening for prostate cancer risk calculator. Eur Urol Open Sci. 2022;41:45–54.
83. Sooriakumaran P, Calaway A, Sagalovich D, Roy S, Srivastava A, Joneja J, et al. The impact of multiple biopsies on outcomes of nerve-sparing robotic-assisted radical prostatectomy. Int J Impot Res. 2012;24(4):161–4.
84. Olvera-Posada D, Welk B, McClure JA, Winick-Ng J, Izawa JI, Pautler SE. The impact of multiple prostate biopsies on risk for major complications following radical prostatectomy: a population-based cohort study. Urology. 2017;106:125–32.
85. Smith DL, Jellison FC, Heldt JP, Tenggardjaja C, Bowman RJ, Jin DH, et al. Robot-assisted radical prostatectomy in patients with previous renal transplantation. J Endourol. 2011;25(10):1643–7.
86. Jhaveri JK, Tan GY, Scherr DS, Tewari AK. Robot-assisted laparoscopic radical prostatectomy in the renal allograft transplant recipient. J Endourol. 2008;22(11):2475–9.
87. Polcari AJ, Allen JC, Nunez-Nateras R, Mmeje CO, Andrews PE, Milner JE, et al. Multicenter experience with robot-assisted radical prostatectomy in renal transplant recipients. Urology. 2012;80(6):1267–72.
88. Léonard G, Pradère B, Monléon L, Boutin JM, Branchereau J, Karam G, et al. Oncological and postoperative outcomes of robot-assisted laparoscopic radical prostatectomy in renal transplant recipients: a multicenter and comparative study. Transplant Proc. 2020;52(3):850–6.
89. Felber M, Drouin SJ, Grande P, Vaessen C, Parra J, Barrou B, et al. Morbidity, perioperative outcomes and complications of robot-assisted radical prostatectomy in kidney transplant patients: a French multicentre study. Urol Oncol. 2020;38(6):599.e15-.e21:599.e15.
90. Pariser JJ, Pearce SM, Patel SG, Bales GT. National trends of simple prostatectomy for benign prostatic hyperplasia with an analysis of risk factors for adverse perioperative outcomes. Urology. 2015;86(4):721–5.
91. Chughtai BI, Simma-Chiang V, Lee R, Isaacs A, Te AE, Kaplan SA, et al. Trends and utilization of laser prostatectomy in ambulatory surgical procedures for the treatment of benign prostatic hyperplasia in New York state (2000-2011). J Endourol. 2015;29(6):700–6.

92. Razdan S. Challenging case: robot-assisted laparoscopic prostatectomy after prior suprapubic open prostatectomy. J Endourol Case Rep. 2018;4(1):72–4.
93. Tsui JF, Feuerstein M, Jazayeri SB, Samadi DB. Robotic assisted laparoscopic prostatectomy performed after previous suprapubic prostatectomy. Case Rep Med. 2016;2016:4573819.

Postoperative Measures to Optimize Early Return of Erectile Function and Urinary Continence

9

Shirin Razdan

Erectile Dysfunction

Background

Post-prostatectomy erectile dysfunction (ED) is reported to be as common as 10–46% at 12 months and 6–37% at 24 months post-robotic-assisted radical prostatectomy (RARP) [1–3]. There are plenty of data supporting degree of nerve sparing and extent of return of erectile dysfunction. Potency rates within 3–24 months after RARP ranged from 29% to 80% with unilateral nerve sparing and 44–93% with bilateral nerve sparing [4]. The mechanism of ED is multifactorial, with both neurogenic and vasculogenic components.

The pelvic plexus is located in the posterolateral wall of the prostate and has been shown to be composed of both parasympathetic and sympathetic tracts that provide autonomic innervation to the corpora cavernosa. Direct injury or thermal injury to these nerves and their terminal branches of the cavernosal nerves during RALP can lead to varying degrees of ED. Additionally, Mulhall et al. showed that in a subset of men with ED post-RALP, they had evidence of venous leak and arteriogenic ED. [5] The theory behind this is that the vascular changes associated with prostatectomy may theoretically induce a hypoxic environment, which may cause cytokine release resulting in cavernosal fibrosis. Additionally, previous studies advocated that neuropraxia can cause long-term low oxygen tension state in the flaccid penis, possibly resulting in smooth muscle apoptosis and fibrosis [6, 7]. These irreversible changes can produce veno-occlusive disruption and venous leak [8].

S. Razdan (✉)
Miami Robotic Surgery at the Comprehensive Urologic Surgery Institute, Miami, FL, USA

S. Razdan, S. Razdan (eds.), *Urinary Continence and Sexual Function After Robotic Prostatectomy, Radiation, and Novel Therapies*,
https://doi.org/10.1007/978-3-031-64245-6_9

Erectile Function

A preoperative patient counseling on the expectations post-RALP is the most important part of physician-patient relationship. Patients should understand that recovery from postoperative erectile function may take up to years and often will not be the same as preoperative function even when maximally attained. Additional sexual changes should be clarified by the urologist, such as reduced libido, changes in orgasm, anejaculation, climacturia, and reduction of penile size [9]. Penile rehabilitation after RALP has become an established therapy for all men with preserved preoperative erectile function undergoing surgery [10]. Studies have shown that early incorporation of penile rehabilitation (<6 months post prostatectomy) results in improved IIEF-EF domain scores when compared with late incorporation of penile rehabilitation (>6 months) [11]. As such, many practitioners now recommend starting medical therapy for ED immediately after catheter removal.

Peer Support

Adherence to any postoperative penile rehabilitation program requires a combination of medical and psychosocial therapy. In this regard, encouraging men to engage in peer support with other men who have undergone RALP plays a big role in postoperative care. Patient testimonials, support groups, and online and social media resources can help demystify some of the expectations and uncertainties of ED after RALP. The treating urologist should guide this discussion; however, recent data has shown that not all online resources, especially those on popular social media sites, are of the same quality [12].

A randomized controlled trial involving 189 heterosexual couples, where the men underwent radical prostatectomy for prostate cancer, showed that men in usual care group had lower unmet sexual supportive care needs than men in the peer and nurse support groups [13]. Partners of those men also described improved sexual adjustment when engaged in peer support rather than in nurse support and usual care [13]. This suggests that there is a role for engagement of both patient and partner with postoperative couples counseling and sexual support groups to improve expected sexual outcomes.

Canada et al. reported that sexual counseling intervention, entailing education on prostate carcinoma and sexual function and options to treat ED as well as sexual communication and stimulation skills, resulted in statistically significant improvement in overall distress among men at 3 months postradical prostatectomy [14]. Intervention also increased both male and female global sexual function at 3 months follow-up, with a return to baseline conditions at 6-month evaluation [14]. As men regained the confidence to engage in sexual activities, they reported an increase of ED medical treatment use from 31% at baseline to 49% at 6-month follow-up [14].

Pelvic Floor Muscle Therapy

Recruitment of levator ani and pelvic floor is a known mechanism for maintaining urinary continence in the post-prostatectomy setting. However, the role of the pelvic floor in the stimulation and maintenance of erections is less clear, although there are theories regarding its utility. During erection, the bulbospongiosus and ischiocavernosus muscles contract and increase penile pressure. Strong contraction of these muscles during intercourse drives more blood into the penis and further increases penile pressure during erection [15]. Training the pelvic floor muscles, with particular focus on the muscles recruited in erection, may be valuable in rehabilitation [16].

Few studies have been performed specifically exploring the utility of pelvic floor muscle therapy (PFMT) in return of erectile function post-RALP. A recent systematic review identified nine such studies and was unable to identify an overwhelming consensus on its utility [17]. This was because different protocols were used in most trials, thereby limiting conclusions. PFMT exercises were either supervised by a trained physical therapist or nurse or were patient directed. The duration and quality of exercises also differed between trials. PFMT has been combined with penile vibratory stimulation, electrostimulation, and biofeedback [16, 18–20].

The combination of PFMT with penile vibratory stimulation did not reach statistical significance, but two trials described combination therapy with electrostimulation and showed improvement in IIEF-EF mean score, although no difference was found between PFMT monotherapy and PFMT with electrostimulation [19, 20]. Biofeedback has the added benefit of teaching subjects to be aware of pelvic floor muscle contraction to promote accurate performance of prescribed exercises. This is performed either through digital rectal examination or anal electromyography [16]. Indeed, studies have shown faster return of erectile function with the addition of biofeedback to PFMT [16].

PDE5is

As a response to sexual stimuli, nitric oxide (NO) is released from endothelial cells in the corpus cavernosum. NO activates the enzyme guanylate cyclase to convert guanosine triphosphate (GTP) into cyclic guanosine monophosphate (cGMP). Accumulation of cGMP leads to smooth muscle relaxation within the corpus cavernosum and increased blood flow to the penis. Phosphodiesterase 5 (PDE5) is an enzyme that converts cGMP to 5′-guanosine monophosphate (5’-GMP). PDE5 inhibitors (PDE5is) competitively inhibit PDE5, enhancing the effects of NO. [21]

PDE5is are the most commonly used medical adjunct in penile rehabilitation programs post-RALP. They are minimally invasive, and patients often tolerate well, with reported side effects including headache, flushing, nasal congestion, nasopharyngitis, and dyspepsia. Mulhall et al. examined the rate of erectile function recovery with PDE5i use post-prostatectomy. They found that men taking one tadalafil (22.3%) daily had achieved “back-to-baseline” IIEF-EF twice as often when compared with as needed (prn) tadalafil (11.8%) and placebo (7.8%) [22]. An animal study involving rats that underwent prostatectomy showed that long-term PDE5i use significantly decreased the amount of smooth muscle cell apoptosis and collagen deposition in corpora cavernosa, corpus spongiosum, and tunica [23]. This suggests that post prostatectomy ED may not simply be due to acute denervation but rather chronic tissue remodeling that can be partially delayed by PDE5i therapy [23].

A systematic review of various post-prostatectomy penile rehabilitation regimens was performed in 2021, and only pelvic floor muscle training (OR 5.21, 95%

CrI 1.24–29.8) and 100 mg sildenafil regular doses, i.e., once daily or nightly (OR 4.00, 95% CrI 1.40–13.4) were associated with a significantly higher likelihood of erectile function recovery [24]. Further research has been done comparing scheduled PDE5i use to on-demand use. Pavlovich et al. compared nightly sildenafil 50 mg with on-demand sildenafil and found no difference at 1 year in erectile recovery between the two groups [25]. Their findings were corroborated by a subsequent randomized controlled trial [26]. This is in contradistinction to the REACTT trial, which compared post-nerve sparing RP daily tadalafil with on-demand and placebo. The authors found that one daily tadalafil 5 mg and on-demand tadalafil 20 mg had improvements in IIEF-EF outcomes in head to head comparison, but daily tadalafil was the only treatment that resulted in significant improvement compared with placebo [27]. Daily tadalafil also had the benefit of decreasing penile length loss at 9 months compared with placebo [27]. Tian et al. in a meta-analysis suggested that daily tadalafil use is preferred in the initial 6 months postoperatively; however, both on-demand and daily PDE5i use can be utilized thereafter to improve objective erectile function parameters [28].

ICI

Intracavernosal injection (ICI) therapy has been long accepted as a treatment option for erectile dysfunction refractory to oral medications. The most common administered drugs are phentolamine, prostaglandin E1 (PGE1), and papaverine. Phentolamine is an alpha-adrenergic antagonist that causes a decrease in peripheral vascular resistance and vasodilatation. PGE1 is an endogenous prostaglandin that elicits cAMP production and thus decreases the influx of calcium within the penile vascular smooth muscle, leading to relaxation of trabecular smooth muscle, arterial dilation, blood entrapment, and erection. Papaverine is a smooth muscle relaxant, causing the nonselective inhibition of PDE enzyme and direct inhibition of calcium channels [4].

Beyond the realm of ED treatment, ICI has also been explored for penile rehabilitation after radical prostatectomy. Montorsi et al. were the first to describe this in 1997. Patients were given ICI of alprostadil three times per week for 6 months and compared with patients without injections. Sixty-seven percent of men that received ICI reported spontaneous erections sufficient for intercourse, while 20% of men in the control group had spontaneous erections [29]. Mulhall et al. also compared men who underwent penile rehab with ICI post-RP to those who did not follow a penile rehab protocol and found an increase in the proportion of men who were able to have intercourse without the use of medication (52% vs. 19%, respectively); mean erectile rigidity (53 ± 21% vs. 26 ± 43%, respectively); mean IIEF-EF (22 ± 6 vs. 12 ± 14, respectively); and response to ICI (95% vs. 76%, respectively) at 18 months post-RP [30].

Intraurethral Suppository

The most commonly used intraurethral suppository is alprostadil (PGE1), which, as previously described, functions by decreasing influx of calcium within the penile vascular smooth muscle, causing smooth muscle relaxation and arterial dilation.

The only randomized controlled trial comparing intraurethral alprostadil (MUSE) for penile rehabilitation after RP compared it with sildenafil and found no difference in spontaneous erectile function at 1 year [31]. Conversely, Raina et al. found that when used as monotherapy, MUSE resulted in 37% more men achieving erections sufficient for intercourse at 6 months, when compared with placebo. Moreover, men in the treatment group had higher sexual health inventory for men (18.9) when compared with the control group (15.8) [32].

Vacuum Erection Devices

Vacuum erection devices (VEDs) mimic an erection using negative pressure to passively engorge the corpora cavernosa. Studies in rats undergoing cavernous nerve injury demonstrated that VED therapy encourages EF recovery after RP by acting on the preservation of both smooth muscle and endothelial integrity via anti-hypoxia, anti-apoptosis, and antifibrotic mechanisms [33]. An additional benefit that may result with daily use of a VED is the preservation of penile length after prostatectomy [33].

A study by Raina et al. showed that in 109 patients who developed ED after nerve-sparing RP, 17% were able to attain spontaneous erections at 9 months with daily use of VEDs, compared with 10% using placebo [34]. On the contrary, a study by Basal et al. showed that VED monotherapy did not improve postoperative erectile function recovery compared with PDE5i monotherapy or PDE5i and VED combination therapy [35]. The most common side effects of VED are mild and include penile numbness, pain, penile bruising, or petechiae. Most of these side effects can be obviated by proper selection of negative pressure. Some men may also endorse sensation of a "cold" penis or glans due to preferential sequestration of venous blood rather than arterial blood from negative pressure [33].

Hyperbaric Oxygen Therapy

Hyperbaric oxygen therapy (HBOT) exposes patients to 100% oxygen at two to three atmospheres, leading to elevated blood-oxygen gradients, which induce stem cell differentiation and in turn lead to neovascularization [36]. Its use has been explored in various clinical scenarios from wound healing to treatment of refractory hemorrhagic cystitis and to acceleration of tissue graft uptake. HBOT has also been compared with placebo treatment in erectile function recovery after nerve sparing radical prostatectomy. Chiles et al. found no significant difference in erectile function scores (as measured by IIEF) at 18 months [37]. As such, HBOT is not currently a recommended treatment option for acceleration of erectile recovery post-RP.

Combination Therapy

The aforementioned treatment options for erectile dysfunction can be used alone or in combination as part of any penile rehabilitation program. Different urologists have different preferred methods of promoting early return of erectile function post-radical prostatectomy. Studies have shown that combination therapy can help with dose reduction and minimizing side effect profile. Nandipati et al. showed that early combination therapy of daily sildenafil with Trimix (compounded phentolamine, alprostadil, and papaverine) resulted in faster return of natural erections and patient satisfaction, with dose reduction of Trimix, minimizing penile pain [38].

Recommendations

For patients with normal preoperative erectile function, urologists should consider minimally invasive penile rehabilitation protocols such as concomitant use of PDE5i and VED as first-line options [39]. PFMT with or without biofeedback should also be routinely incorporated, given its dual benefit on return of erectile function and urinary continence. More invasive procedures such as ICI or intraurethral suppositories and their combination with VED can be offered as second choices [39]. PDE5i monotherapy can be started as early as at the time of catheter removal, given its noninvasive method of administration. Due to their more invasive nature, VED and ICI should be started at least 1 month after the surgery. The frequency of penile rehabilitation should be discussed with each patient's urologist and must balance treatment efficacy with side effects.

Urinary Incontinence

Background

Post-prostatectomy urinary incontinence (PPI) is a devastating side effect of radical prostatectomy. Although most patients (68%) become completely continent within 2 months, persistent urinary incontinence after RP is common and affects 8–25% of patients [40–42]. The robotic approach (RALP) has anecdotally mitigated some of the frequency of this adverse event, allowing for more precise dissection and preservation of the rhabdosphincter, urethral length preservation, and more precise suturing of the anastomosis. A meta-analysis of studies reporting on PPI after RALP by Ficarra et al., showed mean continence rates of 65%, 88%, 91%, and 95% at 3, 6, 12, and 24–36 months, respectively [43]. In spite of this, statistically significant improvement in urinary outcomes has not been seen over the past decade with change in operative approach [44]. Risk factors for PPI include age 65 years or older, high body mass index (BMI), other medical comorbidities, preoperative lower urinary tract symptoms (LUTS), and preoperative urinary incontinence [42, 43].

The challenge in describing outcomes of urinary continence therapy is the variety of ways continence can be described, both subjectively and objectively. Even when relying on quantitative measurement, there is not insignificant variation in describing the incidence and severity of PPI. For example, questionnaire-derived data 12 months after RALP showed a 68% pad-free continence rate [45]. In contrast, when videourodynamics were used, stress urinary incontinence (SUI) was noted in 95% of men at 4 years after RP [46]. The discrepancy between the data provided by these two apparently objective measurements poses a challenge in patient counseling and outcomes research. Moreover, quantitating severity of PPI does not take into account the effect on quality of life, a perhaps more significant metric for patients post-RALP [47].

Urinary Continence

Counseling patients on the urinary outcomes of RALP represents a highly litigious part of the preoperative consent process; thus, the urologist must take their time in explaining the causes of incontinence and set realistic expectations on when patients may regain voluntary bladder control. Additionally, the interplay between urinary continence and sexual activity must be discussed. Climacturia, or leakage during orgasm, affects 28–44% of men who are sexually active after prostatectomy [48]. When stratified by frequency of climacturia, 16% of men experience leakage with every orgasm and 77% "occasionally or rarely." [49] Indeed, up to one third of men who do not report SUI still experience bother from incontinence during sexual activity [50, 51]. The types of and contributors to urinary incontinence include SUI, urgency urinary incontinence (UUI) from overactive bladder (OAB), bladder outlet obstruction (BOO), and underactive bladder. Postoperative measures to hasten return of continence mainly address the loss of sphincteric integrity and subsequent SUI.

PFMT

The most well-established postoperative therapy to stimulate early return of urinary continence post-prostatectomy is pelvic floor muscle therapy (PFMT) [52]. The mechanism of action of PFMT is a gradual strengthening of outlet resistance to the external sphincter and recruitment of other pelvic muscle groups to augment this resistance. There have been multiple different therapy protocols described in the literature as well as varying degrees of supervision. A recent systematic review and meta-analysis of PFMT after radical prostatectomy found a significant benefit of 25% in months 3–6 and 12% at more than 6 months when compared with no PFMT [53]. The authors also found that supervised PFMT resulted in a significant benefit of 16% (1%, 30%) in months three through six post-prostatectomy, but no significant benefit before or after that time frame [53]. Supervised PFMT entailed guidance by a trained nurse or physiotherapist. Another systematic review supported these findings and strongly recommended supervision by a trained specialist to ensure proper muscle contraction and prevent recruitment of abdominal muscles instead of pelvic muscles [54].

The duration of therapy has also been explored. Chitre et al. showed that over time, objective strength of pelvic floor contraction improved, suggesting that continuous practice is needed to maximize pelvic muscle strength [55]. Goode et al. determined that at least 8 weeks of PFMT are necessary to see significant improvement in continence rates [56]. Adjunct therapies such as pilates has also been studied, with no significant additional benefit to PFMT found [57]. Concurrent biofeedback has shown mixed outcomes results, with some studies showing increased enthusiasm of the participant in PFMT when coupled with biofeedback [56, 58].

Recommendations

Pelvic floor muscle therapy should be ubiquitously started in all post-RALP patients with a minimum duration of 8 weeks and continued for at least 6 months. Supervision with a trained physical therapist or nurse helps improve the quality of PFMT and results in improved outcomes. There is no strong evidence in favor of or against concurrent biofeedback.

Conclusion

Erectile dysfunction and urinary incontinence are two of the most devastating consequences of robotic radical prostatectomy. There are, however, numerous postoperative techniques that can be utilized to hasten the return of both functional parameters. Penile rehabilitation with PDE5is and pelvic floor muscle therapy should be started empirically in all men undergoing RALP, with no delay in inception of therapy.

Take-Home Message
Much like prehab, early and aggressive incorporation of postoperative measures to enhance early return of urinary continence and erectile function should be the standard of care for men undergoing radical prostatectomy. There is a large armamentarium of tools and techniques available, and different therapies can be started in a staggered or concurrent manner. Oftentimes, combination therapy encompassing peer support, PFMT, as well as medications is utilized to target the erectile complex as well as accessory continence mechanisms (pelvic floor, striated sphincter).

References

1. Ficarra V, Novara G, Ahlering TE, et al. Systematic review and meta-analysis of studies reporting potency rates after robot-assisted radical prostatectomy. Eur Urol. 2012;62:418.
2. Kim SC, Song C, Kim W, et al. Factors determining functional outcomes after radical prostatectomy: robot-assisted versus retropubic. Eur Urol. 2011;60:413.
3. Krambeck AE, DiMarco DS, Rangel LJ, et al. Radical prostatectomy for prostatic adenocarcinoma: a matched comparison of open retropubic and robot-assisted techniques. BJU Int. 2009;103:448.
4. Lima TFN, Bitran J, Frech FS, et al. Prevalence of post-prostatectomy erectile dysfunction and a review of the recommended therapeutic modalities. Int J Impot Res. 2021;33:401.
5. Mulhall JP, Slovick R, Hotaling J, et al. Erectile dysfunction after radical prostatectomy: hemodynamic profiles and their correlation with the recovery of erectile function. J Urol. 2002;167:1371.

6. Moreland RB. Is there a role of hypoxemia in penile fibrosis: a viewpoint presented to the Society for the Study of Impotence. Int J Impot Res. 1998;10:113.
7. Kim N, Vardi Y, Padma-Nathan H, et al. Oxygen tension regulates the nitric oxide pathway. Physiological role in penile erection. J Clin Invest. 1993;91:437.
8. Lue TF, Tanagho EA. Physiology of erection and pharmacological management of impotence. J Urol. 1987;137:829.
9. Salonia A, Adaikan G, Buvat J, et al. Sexual rehabilitation after treatment for prostate cancer-part 2: recommendations from the fourth international consultation for sexual medicine (ICSM 2015). J Sex Med. 2017;14:297.
10. Jo JK, Jeong SJ, Oh JJ, et al. Effect of starting penile rehabilitation with sildenafil immediately after robot-assisted laparoscopic radical prostatectomy on erectile function recovery: a prospective randomized trial. J Urol. 2018;199:1600.
11. Mulhall JP, Parker M, Waters BW, et al. The timing of penile rehabilitation after bilateral nerve-sparing radical prostatectomy affects the recovery of erectile function. BJU Int. 2010;105:37.
12. Dubin JM, Aguiar JA, Lin JS, et al. The broad reach and inaccuracy of men's health information on social media: analysis of TikTok and Instagram. Int J Impot Res. 2022;1:256–60.
13. Chambers SK, Occhipinti S, Stiller A, et al. Five-year outcomes from a randomised controlled trial of a couples-based intervention for men with localised prostate cancer. Psychooncology. 2019;28:775.
14. Canada AL, Neese LE, Sui D, et al. Pilot intervention to enhance sexual rehabilitation for couples after treatment for localized prostate carcinoma. Cancer. 2005;104:2689.
15. Dorey G. Conservative treatment of erectile dysfunction. 3: literature review. Br J Nurs. 2000;9:859.
16. Prota C, Gomes CM, Ribeiro LH, et al. Early postoperative pelvic-floor biofeedback improves erectile function in men undergoing radical prostatectomy: a prospective, randomized, controlled trial. Int J Impot Res. 2012;24:174.
17. Wong C, Louie DR, Beach C. A systematic review of pelvic floor muscle training for erectile dysfunction after prostatectomy and recommendations to guide further research. J Sex Med. 2020;17:737.
18. Fode M, Borre M, Ohl DA, et al. Penile vibratory stimulation in the recovery of urinary continence and erectile function after nerve-sparing radical prostatectomy: a randomized, controlled trial. BJU Int. 2014;114:111.
19. Geraerts I, Van Poppel H, Devoogdt N, et al. Pelvic floor muscle training for erectile dysfunction and climacturia 1 year after nerve sparing radical prostatectomy: a randomized controlled trial. Int J Impot Res. 2016;28:9.
20. Laurienzo CE, Magnabosco WJ, Jabur F, et al. Pelvic floor muscle training and electrical stimulation as rehabilitation after radical prostatectomy: a randomized controlled trial. J Phys Ther Sci. 2018;30:825.
21. Huang SA, Lie JD. Phosphodiesterase-5 (PDE5) inhibitors in the management of erectile dysfunction. P T. 2013;38:407.
22. Mulhall JP, Brock G, Oelke M, et al. Effects of tadalafil once-daily or on-demand vs placebo on return to baseline erectile function after bilateral nerve-sparing radical prostatectomy – results from a randomized controlled trial (REACTT). J Sex Med. 2016;13:679.
23. Kovanecz I, Rambhatla A, Ferrini M, et al. Long-term continuous sildenafil treatment ameliorates corporal veno-occlusive dysfunction (CVOD) induced by cavernosal nerve resection in rats. Int J Impot Res. 2008;20:202.
24. Sari Motlagh R, Abufaraj M, Yang L, et al. Penile rehabilitation strategy after nerve sparing radical prostatectomy: a systematic review and network meta-analysis of randomized trials. J Urol. 2021;205:1018.
25. Pavlovich CP, Levinson AW, Su LM, et al. Nightly vs on-demand sildenafil for penile rehabilitation after minimally invasive nerve-sparing radical prostatectomy: results of a randomized double-blind trial with placebo. BJU Int. 2013;112:844.

26. Kim DJ, Hawksworth DJ, Hurwitz LM, et al. A prospective, randomized, placebo-controlled trial of on-demand vs. nightly sildenafil citrate as assessed by Rigiscan and the international index of erectile function. Andrology. 2016;4:27.
27. Montorsi F, Brock G, Stolzenburg JU, et al. Effects of tadalafil treatment on erectile function recovery following bilateral nerve-sparing radical prostatectomy: a randomised placebo-controlled study (REACTT). Eur Urol. 2014;65:587.
28. Tian D, Wang XY, Zong HT, et al. Efficacy and safety of short- and long-term, regular and on-demand regimens of phosphodiesterase type 5 inhibitors in treating erectile dysfunction after nerve-sparing radical prostatectomy: a systematic review and meta-analysis. Clin Interv Aging. 2017;12:405.
29. Montorsi F, Guazzoni G, Strambi LF, et al. Recovery of spontaneous erectile function after nerve-sparing radical retropubic prostatectomy with and without early intracavernous injections of alprostadil: results of a prospective, randomized trial. J Urol. 1997;158:1408.
30. Mulhall J, Land S, Parker M, et al. The use of an erectogenic pharmacotherapy regimen following radical prostatectomy improves recovery of spontaneous erectile function. J Sex Med. 2005;2:532.
31. McCullough AR, Hellstrom WG, Wang R, et al. Recovery of erectile function after nerve sparing radical prostatectomy and penile rehabilitation with nightly intraurethral alprostadil versus sildenafil citrate. J Urol. 2010;183:2451.
32. Raina R, Pahlajani G, Agarwal A, et al. The early use of transurethral alprostadil after radical prostatectomy potentially facilitates an earlier return of erectile function and successful sexual activity. BJU Int. 2007;100:1317.
33. Lehrfeld T, Lee DI. The role of vacuum erection devices in penile rehabilitation after radical prostatectomy. Int J Impot Res. 2009;21:158.
34. Raina R, Agarwal A, Ausmundson S, et al. Early use of vacuum constriction device following radical prostatectomy facilitates early sexual activity and potentially earlier return of erectile function. Int J Impot Res. 2006;18:77.
35. Basal S, Wambi C, Acikel C, et al. Optimal strategy for penile rehabilitation after robot-assisted radical prostatectomy based on preoperative erectile function. BJU Int. 2013;111:658.
36. Ortega MA, Fraile-Martinez O, García-Montero C, et al. A general overview on the hyperbaric oxygen therapy: applications, mechanisms and translational opportunities. Medicina (Kaunas). 2021;57:864.
37. Chiles KA, Staff, I, Johnson-Arbor K, et al. A double-blind, randomized trial on the efficacy and safety of hyperbaric oxygenation therapy in the preservation of erectile function after radical prostatectomy. J Urol. 2018;199:805.
38. Nandipati K, Raina R, Agarwal A, et al. Early combination therapy: intracavernosal injections and sildenafil following radical prostatectomy increases sexual activity and the return of natural erections. Int J Impot Res. 2006;18:446.
39. Segal RL, Bivalacqua TJ, Burnett AL. Current penile-rehabilitation strategies: clinical evidence. Arab J Urol. 2013;11:230.
40. Majoros A, Bach D, Keszthelyi A, et al. Urinary incontinence and voiding dysfunction after radical retropubic prostatectomy (prospective urodynamic study). Neurourol Urodyn. 2006;25:2.
41. Potosky AL, Davis WW, Hoffman RM, et al. Five-year outcomes after prostatectomy or radiotherapy for prostate cancer: the prostate cancer outcomes study. J Natl Cancer Inst. 2004;96:1358.
42. Holm HV, Fosså SD, Hedlund H, et al. How should continence and incontinence after radical prostatectomy be evaluated? A prospective study of patient ratings and changes with time. J Urol. 2014;192:1155.
43. Ficarra V, Novara G, Rosen RC, et al. Systematic review and meta-analysis of studies reporting urinary continence recovery after robot-assisted radical prostatectomy. Eur Urol. 2012;62:405.
44. Clements MB, Gmelich CC, Vertosick EA, et al. Have urinary function outcomes after radical prostatectomy improved over the past decade? Cancer. 2022;128:1066.

45. Wiltz AL, Shikanov S, Eggener SE, et al. Robotic radical prostatectomy in overweight and obese patients: oncological and validated-functional outcomes. Urology. 2009;73:316.
46. Kielb SJ, Clemens JQ. Comprehensive urodynamics evaluation of 146 men with incontinence after radical prostatectomy. Urology. 2005;66:392.
47. Trofimenko V, Myers JB, Brant WO. Post-prostatectomy incontinence: how common and bothersome is it really? Sex Med Rev. 2017;5:536.
48. O'Neil BB, Presson A, Gannon J, et al. Climacturia after definitive treatment of prostate cancer. J Urol. 2014;191:159.
49. Barnas JL, Pierpaoli S, Ladd P, et al. The prevalence and nature of orgasmic dysfunction after radical prostatectomy. BJU Int. 2004;94:603.
50. Guay A, Seftel AD. Sexual foreplay incontinence in men with erectile dysfunction after radical prostatectomy: a clinical observation. Int J Impot Res. 2008;20:199.
51. Mitchell SA, Jain RK, Laze J, et al. Post-prostatectomy incontinence during sexual activity: a single center prevalence study. J Urol. 2011;186:982.
52. Van Kampen M, De Weerdt W, Van Poppel H, et al. Effect of pelvic-floor re-education on duration and degree of incontinence after radical prostatectomy: a randomised controlled trial. Lancet. 2000;355:98.
53. Baumann FT, Reimer N, Gockeln T, et al. Supervised pelvic floor muscle exercise is more effective than unsupervised pelvic floor muscle exercise at improving urinary incontinence in prostate cancer patients following radical prostatectomy – a systematic review and meta-analysis. Disabil Rehabil. 2022;44:5374.
54. Park JJ, Kwon A, Park JY, et al. Efficacy of pelvic floor exercise for post-prostatectomy incontinence: systematic review and meta-analysis. Urology. 2022;168:175.
55. Chitre A, Kulkarni JN. Effect of early pelvic floor muscle exercises (Kegel's) after robotic prostatectomy in prostate cancer patients. J Robot Surg. 2022;17:1065.
56. Goode PS, Burgio KL, Johnson TM 2nd, et al. Behavioral therapy with or without biofeedback and pelvic floor electrical stimulation for persistent postprostatectomy incontinence: a randomized controlled trial. JAMA. 2011;305:151.
57. Gomes CS, Pedriali FR, Urbano MR, et al. The effects of Pilates method on pelvic floor muscle strength in patients with post-prostatectomy urinary incontinence: a randomized clinical trial. Neurourol Urodyn. 2018;37:346.
58. An D, Wang J, Zhang F, et al. Effects of biofeedback combined with Pilates training on post-prostatectomy incontinence. Urology. 2021;155:152.

Urinary Continence and Erectile Function in the Salvage Setting

10

Marcio Covas Moschovas, Evan Patel, David Loy, and Vipul Patel

Introduction

Robotic surgery has expanded in the last 20 years since the first robot was released to the market in 2000 [1, 2]. In this scenario, robotic-assisted radical prostatectomy (RARP) became the most common procedure performed by urologists with access to this technology worldwide [3, 4]. However, even with these technological advancements, other types of less-invasive therapies have been described to treat patients with prostate cancer, including radiation therapy (RT) [5, 6] and several techniques of focal therapy (FT) [7, 8].

With all these approaches available in clinical management, patients have a wide range of different treatments for localized tumors in prostate cancer. However, the most challenging scenario concerns PSA recurrence in patients who did primary nonsurgical treatments, such as RT and FT. In these cases, the salvage robotic-assisted radical prostatectomy (S-RARP) is an option for patients who do not want to repeat RT or FT in these salvage settings.

S-RARP is always challenging for surgeons and patients due to the lack of anatomical landmarks, disease aggressiveness after recurrence, and suboptimal functional and oncological outcomes. In this chapter, we will describe the technical details and current status of continence and potency recovery outcomes following salvage robotic-assisted radical prostatectomy.

M. C. Moschovas (✉) · V. Patel
AdventHealth Global Robotics Institute, Celebration, FL, USA

University of Central Florida (UCF), Orlando, FL, USA
e-mail: Vipul.patel.md@adventhealth.com

E. Patel · D. Loy
AdventHealth Global Robotics Institute, Celebration, FL, USA

S. Razdan, S. Razdan (eds.), *Urinary Continence and Sexual Function After Robotic Prostatectomy, Radiation, and Novel Therapies*,
https://doi.org/10.1007/978-3-031-64245-6_10

Salvage Robotic-Assisted Radical Prostatectomy Literature

Literature Search Strategy

In this chapter, we described in Table 10.1 a systematic literature review of studies reporting S-RARP outcomes in the last 6 years (from January 2016 to June 2022). In articles mixing different approaches, we included only the robotic surgery data on S-RARP and excluded the data of open and laparoscopic. We included the PubMed® databank, searching for all available articles in English using the terms "salvage robotic-assisted radical prostatectomy, salvage robotic laparoscopic prostatectomy, and salvage robotic radical prostatectomy."

Literature Summary

Table 10.1 illustrates the available articles containing S-RARP and all primary treatments performed before surgery, such as radiotherapy (RT), high-intensity focused ultrasound (HIFU), cryotherapy (Cryo), brachytherapy (BRC), external beam radiotherapy (EBRT), and others. However, some of these nonsurgical therapies, such as radiotherapy, can present up to 69% of biochemical recurrence (BCR), and 5–83% of the patients will require further treatment (salvage) after the primary therapy for prostate cancer [8–12].

Overall, we identified 28 articles with a median follow-up that ranges from 7 to 44 months [13–40]. All studies were case series based on retrospective data evaluation. Table 10.1 describes the data collected on each study, including the year of publication, the number of patients in each study, the type of primary therapy, total operative time (TOT), console time (CT), intraoperative complications (IOC), estimated blood loss (EBL), postoperative complications (POC) according to Clavien-Dindo (Clv), positive surgical margins (PSM), continence, potency, biochemical recurrence (BCR), and median follow-up (MFU) in months.

Primary Therapies for Prostate Cancer (PCa) Before S-RARP

In the current literature series, we identified that more than 50% of the patients underwent radiotherapy as a primary treatment before the salvage treatment, and focal therapy was the second most common approach.

Surgical Performance and Complications

The total operative time ranges from 120 to 303 minutes, and the console time ranges from 79 to 199 minutes. The estimated blood loss (EBL) ranges from 50 to 465 ml. Intra- and postoperative complications range from 0 to 9.1% and 0 to 34.9%, respectively (Clv 1 to 4). Rectal injury, one of the most common complications during S-RARP, in the contemporary series, was 0.48% [23].

Table 10.1 The current studies on salvage robotic-assisted radical prostatectomy

Author	Year	N. of patients	Primary therapy	TOT/CT (minutes)	IOC (%)	EBL (ml)	POC (Clavien) In 90 days (%)	PSM (%)	Continence/ potency (%)	BCR (%)	MFU months
Vora [13]	2016	6	RT	NA/NA	0	NA	16.7	NA	83.4/NA	16.7	7.2
Kenney [14]	2016	20	RT	303/NA	5	381	30 Clv ≥3	15	NA/NA	22	9.5
Ozu C [15]	2016	1	HIRT	244/189	0	100	0	0	NA/NA	0	10
Orré M [16]	2017	7	BRC	148/NA	0	NA	14 Clv ≥3	14	50/66	14	24
Ou YC [17]	2017	14	RT-11 CKR-2 HIFU-1	NA/134	7	99	21	21.4	71.4/66.7	21	32.4
Nunes-Silva [18]	2017	22	FT	134/NA	9.1	465	NA	4.5	31/73	31.8	7
Ogaya-Pinies [19]	2017	60	EBRT-35 BRC-10 PB-6 Cryo-7 HIFU-2	131/NA	0	130	5 Clv 1–2	NA	50/NA	NA	12
Bonet X [20]	2018	80	RT-63 ABL-17	NA/NA	NA	NA	NA	NA	53.7/16.6	26.1	22
Ogaya-Pinies [22]	2018	96	EBRT-37 BRC-14 BRC + EBRT-13 CYK-3 PB-1 Cryo-18 HIFU-7 Others 4	125/NA	0	100	26 Clv 1–4	16.7	57.3/54.8	15	14

(continued)

Table 10.1 (continued)

Author	Year	N. of patients	Primary therapy	TOT/CT (minutes)	IOC (%)	EBL (ml)	POC (Clavien) In 90 days (%)	PSM (%)	Continence/ potency (%)	BCR (%)	MFU months
Marconi L [21]	2019	82	HIFU-57 Cryo-16 IRE-4 VTP-3 PRX302–2	NA/NA	0	400	6.1 Clv 1-3b	13.4	83/14	41.5	13
Gontero P [23]	2019	209	RT-121 BRC-55 Cryo-14 HIFU-9 Others-10	228/NA	0.48	222	34.9 Clv1–4	NA	57.5/8.1	NA	28.8
Onol FF [24]	2019	126	RT-94 ABL-32	130/85 120/79	0 0	100 100	20 Clv 1–4 9 Clv 1-3a	17 43.8	51.3/13 87.5/27	17 18	32 29
Thompson JE [25]	2020	45	HIFU	NA/140	0	200	17.8 Clv 1–3	44.4	65.5/???	5.3	17.7
Bonet X [26]	2020	120	RT ABL	127/84	0	103	14.2 Clv1–4	22.5	55.8/19.2	32.5	44
De Groote R [27]	2020	106	HIFU-59 RT-27 BRC-10 Others –10	NA/NA	NA	NA	8	39	50/5	13	25
Madi R [28]	2021	20 Retzius 6 Standard	EBRT-18 BRC-4 Cryo-2 CYK-2	NA/141 NA/199	0 0	50 100	10 Clv 1–3 16.7 Clv 3	30 33	100/NA 44/NA	20 33.3	18
Marra G [29]	2021	198	RT BRC	NA	NA	NA	NA	15.7	NA	19	NA

Cathcart P [30]	2021	23	Cryo (4) HIFU (17) Electro (1)	NA	0	NA	4 (Clv 1)	35	100/52	17.4	12
Martinez PF [31]	2021	26	BRC (3) EBRT (19) IMRT (3)	NA	5 rectal	150	11.5(Clv 3–5)	26.9	90.9/4.5	15	47
Nathan A [32]	2021	135	Focal	165/NA	0	200	13.3 (Clv 1–5)	37.8	78.8/5.2	22.2	43
Nunes-Silva [33]	2021	*RS (12)	EBRT (10) BRC (2)	NA/138	0	81	8.3(Clv 3)	25	91.6%/NA	16.6	12
Kowalczyk K [34]	2021	*RS (40)	EBRT (21) BRC (12) HIFU (7)	NA/130	2.5	100	12.5 (Clv 1–5)	57.5	54.1/10	23.1	23
Kowalczyk K [34]	2021	32	EBRT (16) BRC (9) Cryo (5) RT (2)	NA/175	0	150	28.1(Clv 1–3)	65.6	6.3/12.5	37.5	36
Spitznagel T [35]	2021	13	HIFU	260/NA	0	230	46,2 (Clv 1–3)	7.6	5.1/9.1	7.6	12
Bozkurt Y [36]	2021	10	PTB	230/NA	0	745	90 (Clv 1–4)	20	20/71	10	31.8
Bhat KRS [37]	2021	53	Focal	NA/121	0	100	21 (Clv1–2)	40	56/13	17	36.3
Schuetz V [38]	2021	*RS (21)	RT (8) HIFU (9) BRC (2) Cryo (1) Focal (1)	228/NA	0	300	NA	23.8	19/NA	14.3	12

(continued)

Table 10.1 (continued)

Author	Year	N. of patients	Primary therapy	TOT/CT (minutes)	IOC (%)	EBL (ml)	POC (Clavien) In 90 days (%)	PSM (%)	Continence/ potency (%)	BCR (%)	MFU months
Schuetz V [38]	2021	7	RT (4) HIFU (1) BRC (2)	252/NA	0	500	NA	71.4	0/NA	57.1	36
Blazevski [39]	2022	15	Focal	NA/NA	0	200	NA	7	100/60		22
Mortensen [40]	2022	5	EBRT	205/NA	0	120	3 (Clv 1–2)	75	0/NA	20	13

Clv Clavien-Dindo, *EBL* estimated blood loss, *PSM* positive surgical margins, *TOT* total operative time, *CT* console time, *IOC* intraoperative complication, *POC* postoperative complications, *NA* not available, *MFU* median follow-up, *PB* proton beam, *Cryo* cryotherapy, *CYK* Cyberknife, *BCR* biochemical recurrence, *RT* radiotherapy, *HIRT* heavy iron radiotherapy therapy, *BRC* brachytherapy, *CK* Cyberknife radiation, *HIFU* high-intensity focused ultrasound, *FT* focal therapy, *EBRT* external-beam radiotherapy, *ABL* ablation, *IRE* irreversible electroporation, *VTP* vascular-targeted photodynamic therapy, *PRX302* Topsalysin, *Electro* electroporation, *IMRT* intensity-modulated radiotherapy, *RS Retzius sparing, *PTB* proton beam

Functional Outcomes

When evaluating functional outcomes summary among the series, the data diverge among the centers, and the continence rates range from 31% to 100%, while potency ranges from 0 to 73%. Most articles lack details about radiation dose or type of energy used in FT, and almost all studies do not describe the individual outcome of each therapy.

Pathological and Oncological Outcomes

Positive surgical margins reached up to 44.4%, while biochemical recurrence ranged from 0 to 41.5%. All studies reported BCR according to RTOG-ASTRO Phoenix Criteria [3]. However, BCR in 5 years was not available in most series due to the short-term follow-up of all studies.

Experience and Challenges of S-RARP

In this chapter, we summarized all current series on salvage robotic-assisted radical prostatectomy. Reporting and comparing these outcomes are challenging because all available data is based on retrospective studies with a small number of patients and all its inherent risks of bias. Most studies described the overall S-RARP outcomes adding different primary therapies, without specifying or separating the patients and results according to the primary treatment. Furthermore, the surgeries were performed by several surgeons with diverse levels of expertise and techniques. In addition, most studies failed to report the primary therapy details, such as radiation dose, type of energy used on the focal approach, and side of the primary tumor.

Several factors may influence the postoperative recovery of potency and continence following S-RARP. The first element is patient related and regards the preoperative potency after undergoing a local treatment. Even with less invasive modalities, these therapies have inflammatory impacts on the prostate neural bundles and decrease the basal potency rates of these patients. Therefore, patients with suboptimal potency rates before surgery will have suboptimal erection recovery after S-RARP. Second, the inflammatory process and tissue damage by the primary treatment displace and modify the local anatomy and challenge surgeons while identifying the appropriate anatomical landmarks. Consequently, to maintain oncological principles and minimize positive surgical margins, in some cases, the dissection expands through the endopelvic fascia, apical sphincter, and neural bundles, impacting postoperative potency and continence recovery.

Different therapies usually cause different types of prostate damage according to the tumor's location and the types of energy used. In patients with previous radiation, we typically visualize a fibrotic process in the whole gland, posing a challenging nerve-sparing on both sides. In addition, these patients have intense fibrosis at the apex and bladder neck, which impacts the anastomosis tension and healing

(Fig. 10.1). In our experience, these patients have the worst potency and continence recovery rates [24]. Similarly, in patients with previous brachytherapy, we usually visualize the seeds at the apex and the endopelvic fascia (Fig. 10.2). In these cases, fibrotic tissue is present mainly at the apical portion of the prostate and also impacts the anastomosis healing process and continence recovery. It is important to know when the primary therapy was done because, before 6–10 months, the seeds could still be radioactive with potential harm to the surgical team [41].

The rationale of focal therapy is to perform cancer treatment with minimum injury to the surrounding tissues. However, in our experience, FT also causes contralateral damage, and, in most cases, the contralateral side of the ablation often presents a fibrotic aspect with challenging anatomical landmarks [24, 37]. These patients have better potency and continence recovery compared with patients with

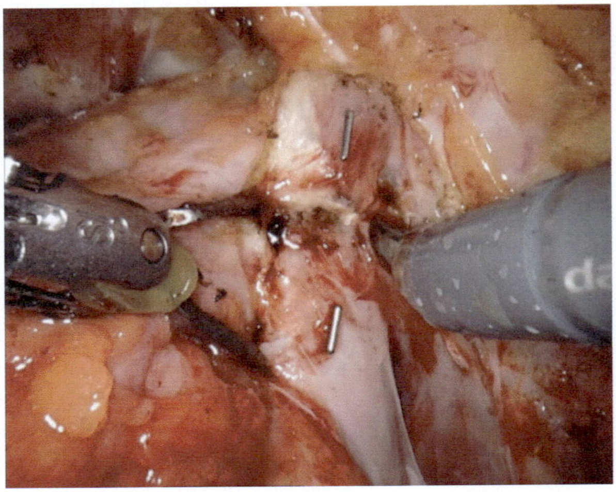

Fig. 10.1 Fibrotic tissue around the prostate

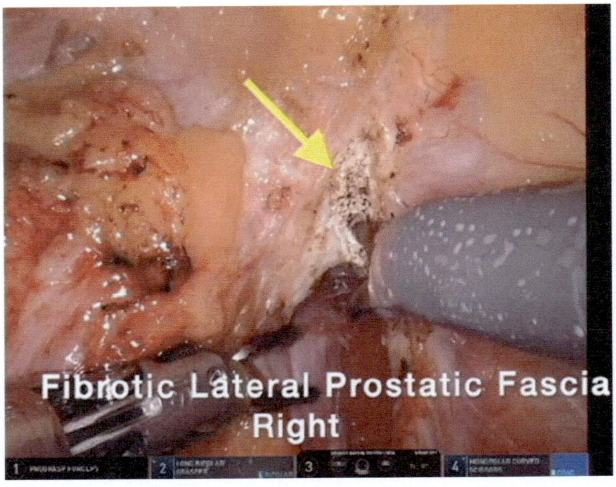

Fig. 10.2 Brachy seeds on the prostate apex

previous RT, but these rates are still suboptimal compared with primary robotic-assisted radical prostatectomy.

Some studies have assessed the S-RARP outcomes of patients selected according to the primary therapy. Two of them reported and compared the results of S-RARP following ablation and radiation. The authors had similar conclusions regarding functional outcomes between the therapies [16, 19, 24, 27]. In both articles, potency and continence rates were higher in patients who underwent primary ablations. Kenney et al. described the S-RARP in patients with previous radiation and complications with Clavien-Dindo ≥3 reached up to 30%, while PSM and BCR reached 15% and 22%, respectively [14]. In another study, Orré M et al. reported 14% of PSM and 14% of BCR in patients with previous brachytherapy [16].

Finally, another challenge regards the expertise with this type of surgery. We believe that it is crucial to have extensive experience with robotic surgery before facing the first salvage surgery because, besides the suboptimal outcomes of potency and continence, the margin rates are crucial to achieving optimal oncological outcomes. In addition, the intra- and postoperative complications are higher with increased rates of rectal injury, especially following proton treatment. We described the learning curve of this surgery in more than 120 cases, and currently with a series of almost 400 salvage robotic-assisted radical prostatectomies, we believe each surgery is unique and each therapy needs an individual surgical approach [26]. Therefore, knowing the details about the primary therapy is crucial for achieving the best results.

Conclusion

Salvage robotic-assisted radical prostatectomy is a challenging procedure for patients and surgeons due to suboptimal outcomes posed by several anatomical and functional modifications after the primary therapy. The current S-RARP studies describe low rates of intraoperative complications and small blood loss. However, potency and continence rates are largely reduced compared with the primary RARP series, and better-designed studies are still needed to assess the long-term results and individually determine the primary therapy impacts on the surgical outcomes. In this scenario, we believe it is crucial to have significant expertise in robotic-assisted radical prostatectomy before facing the first salvage case.

Take-Home Message

This is an important chapter highlighting the suboptimal outcomes and technical challenges of salvage prostatectomy. The authors also comment on specific differences noted at the time of surgery when salvage is performed after external beam radiation, brachytherapy, or focal therapy. Urologists performing salvage prostatectomy should be prepared to encounter tougher dissection planes, globally after EBRT and focally at apex with BT. Focal therapies appear to also cause an inflammatory reaction on the side contralateral to treatment as well and should be anticipated at time of surgery.

Disclosure The authors have no disclosures.

References

1. Sapre N, Shah TT, Dasgupta P. Current and upcoming robotic surgery platforms and adjunctive technologies. In: Robotic urologic surgery. Springer International Publishing; 2022. p. 11–20. https://doi.org/10.1007/978-3-031-00363-9_2.
2. Noël J, Reddy S, Giedelman C, Swarovski-Adams RCD, Patel E, Satava RM. History of robotic surgery. In: Robotic urologic surgery. Springer International Publishing; 2022. p. 3–10. https://doi.org/10.1007/978-3-031-00363-9_1.
3. Mottet N, van den Bergh RCN, Briers E, et al. EAU-EANM-ESTRO-ESUR-SIOG guidelines on prostate cancer—2020 update. Part 1: screening, diagnosis, and local treatment with curative intent. Eur Urol. 2021;79(2):243–62. https://doi.org/10.1016/j.eururo.2020.09.042.
4. Grossman DC, Curry SJ, Owens DK, et al. Screening for prostate cancer. JAMA. 2018;319(18):1901. https://doi.org/10.1001/jama.2018.3710.
5. Valle LF, Lehrer EJ, Markovic D, et al. A systematic review and meta-analysis of local salvage therapies after radiotherapy for prostate cancer (MASTER). Eur Urol. 2021;80(3):280–92. https://doi.org/10.1016/j.eururo.2020.11.010.
6. Wallis CJD, Saskin R, Choo R, et al. Surgery versus radiotherapy for clinically-localized prostate cancer: a systematic review and meta-analysis. Eur Urol. 2016;70(1):21–30. https://doi.org/10.1016/j.eururo.2015.11.010.
7. Abreu AL, Kaneko M, Cacciamani GE, Lebastchi AH. Focal therapy for prostate cancer: getting ready for prime time. Eur Urol. 2022;81(1):34–6. https://doi.org/10.1016/j.eururo.2021.10.005.
8. Valerio M, Cerantola Y, Eggener SE, et al. New and established technology in focal ablation of the prostate: a systematic review. Eur Urol. 2017;71(1):17–34. https://doi.org/10.1016/j.eururo.2016.08.044.
9. Bass R, Fleshner N, Finelli A, Barkin J, Zhang L, Klotz L. Oncologic and functional outcomes of partial gland ablation with high intensity focused ultrasound for localized prostate cancer. J Urol. 2019;201(1):113–9. https://doi.org/10.1016/j.juro.2018.07.040.
10. Martino P, Scattoni V, Galosi AB, et al. Role of imaging and biopsy to assess local recurrence after definitive treatment for prostate carcinoma (surgery, radiotherapy, cryotherapy, HIFU). World J Urol. 2011;29(5):595–605. https://doi.org/10.1007/s00345-011-0687-y.
11. Agarwal PK, Sadetsky N, Konety BR, Resnick MI, Carroll PR, Cancer of the Prostate Strategic Urological Research Endeavor (CaPSURE). Treatment failure after primary and salvage therapy for prostate cancer: likelihood, patterns of care, and outcomes. Cancer. 2008;112(2):307–14. https://doi.org/10.1002/cncr.23161.
12. Roach M, Hanks G, Thames H, et al. Defining biochemical failure following radiotherapy with or without hormonal therapy in men with clinically localized prostate cancer: recommendations of the RTOG-ASTRO Phoenix Consensus Conference. Int J Radiat Oncol Biol Phys. 2006;65(4):965–74. https://doi.org/10.1016/j.ijrobp.2006.04.029.
13. Vora A, Agarwal V, Singh P, et al. Single-institution comparative study on the outcomes of salvage cryotherapy versus salvage robotic prostatectomy for radio-resistant prostate cancer. Prostate Int. 2016;4(1):7–10. https://doi.org/10.1016/j.prnil.2015.11.002.
14. Kenney PA, Nawaf CB, Mustafa M, et al. Robotic-assisted laparoscopic versus open salvage radical prostatectomy following radiotherapy. Can J Urol. 2016;23(3):8271–7.
15. Ozu C, Aoki K, Nakamura K, et al. The initial case report: salvage robotic assisted radical prostatectomy after heavy ion radiotherapy. Urol Case Rep. 2016;7:45–7. https://doi.org/10.1016/j.eucr.2016.04.008.
16. Orré M, Piéchaud T, Sargos P, Richaud P, Roubaud G, Thomas L. Oncological and functional results of robotic salvage radical prostatectomy after permanent brachytherapy implants. Cancer Radiother. 2017;21(2):119–23. https://doi.org/10.1016/j.canrad.2016.11.001.

17. Salvage robotic-assisted laparoscopic radical prostatectomy: experience with 14 cases. Anticancer Res. 2017;37(4):2045–50. https://doi.org/10.21873/anticanres.11550.
18. Nunes-Silva I, Barret E, Srougi V, et al. Effect of prior focal therapy on perioperative, oncologic and functional outcomes of salvage robotic assisted radical prostatectomy. J Urol. 2017;198(5):1069–76. https://doi.org/10.1016/j.juro.2017.05.071.
19. Ogaya-Pinies G, Kadakia Y, Palayapalayam-Ganapathi H, et al. Use of scaffolding tissue biografts to bolster vesicourethral anastomosis during salvage robot-assisted prostatectomy reduces leak rates and catheter times. Eur Urol. 2018;74(1):92–8. https://doi.org/10.1016/j.eururo.2016.10.004.
20. Bonet X, Ogaya-Pinies G, Woodlief T, et al. Nerve-sparing in salvage robot-assisted prostatectomy: surgical technique, oncological and functional outcomes at a single high-volume institution. BJU Int. 2018;122(5):837–44. https://doi.org/10.1111/bju.14517.
21. Marconi L, Stonier T, Tourinho-Barbosa R, et al. Robot-assisted radical prostatectomy after focal therapy: oncological, functional outcomes and predictors of recurrence. Eur Urol. 2019;76(1):27–30. https://doi.org/10.1016/j.eururo.2019.03.007.
22. Ogaya-Pinies G, Linares-Espinos E, Hernandez-Cardona E, et al. Salvage robotic-assisted radical prostatectomy: oncologic and functional outcomes from two high-volume institutions. World J Urol. 2019;37(8):1499–505. https://doi.org/10.1007/s00345-018-2406-4.
23. Gontero P, Marra G, Alessio P, et al. Salvage radical prostatectomy for recurrent prostate cancer: morbidity and functional outcomes from a large multicenter series of open versus robotic approaches. J Urol. 2019;202(4):725–31. https://doi.org/10.1097/JU.0000000000000327.
24. Onol FF, Bhat S, Moschovas M, et al. Comparison of outcomes of salvage robot-assisted laparoscopic prostatectomy for post-primary radiation vs focal therapy. BJU Int. 2020;125(1):103–11. https://doi.org/10.1111/bju.14900.
25. Thompson JE, Sridhar AN, Shaw G, et al. Peri-operative, functional and early oncologic outcomes of salvage robotic-assisted radical prostatectomy after high-intensity focused ultrasound partial ablation. BMC Urol. 2020;20(1):81. https://doi.org/10.1186/s12894-020-00656-9.
26. Bonet X, Moschovas MC, Onol FF, et al. The surgical learning curve for salvage robot-assisted radical prostatectomy: a prospective single-surgeon study. Minerva Urol Nephrol. 2021;73(5):600. https://doi.org/10.23736/S2724-6051.20.04077-1.
27. de Groote R, Nathan A, de Bleser E, et al. Techniques and outcomes of salvage Robot-Assisted Radical Prostatectomy (sRARP). Eur Urol. 2020;78(6):885–92. https://doi.org/10.1016/j.eururo.2020.05.003.
28. Madi R, Sayyid RK, Hiffa A, Thomas E, Terris MK, Klaassen Z. Early experience with salvage Retzius-sparing robotic-assisted radical prostatectomy: oncologic and functional outcomes. Urology. 2021;149:117–21. https://doi.org/10.1016/j.urology.2020.12.029.
29. Marra G, Karnes RJ, Calleris G, et al. Oncological outcomes of salvage radical prostatectomy for recurrent prostate cancer in the contemporary era: a multicenter retrospective study. Urol Oncol. 2021;39(5):296.e21–9. https://doi.org/10.1016/j.urolonc.2020.11.002.
30. Cathcart P, Ribeiro L, Moore C, et al. Outcomes of the RAFT trial: robotic surgery after focal therapy. BJU Int. 2021;128(4):504–10. https://doi.org/10.1111/bju.15432.
31. Martinez PF, Romeo A, Tobia I, Isola M, Giudice CR, Villamil WA. Comparing open and robotic salvage radical prostatectomy after radiotherapy: predictors and outcomes. Prostate Int. 2021;9(1):42–7. https://doi.org/10.1016/j.prnil.2020.07.003.
32. Nathan A, Fricker M, de Groote R, et al. Salvage versus primary robot-assisted radical prostatectomy: a propensity-matched comparative effectiveness study from a high-volume tertiary centre. Eur Urol Open Sci. 2021;27:43–52. https://doi.org/10.1016/j.euros.2021.03.003.
33. Nunes-Silva I, Hidaka AK, Monti CR, Tobias-Machado M, Zampolli H d C. Salvage Retzius sparing robotic assisted radical prostatectomy: the first brazilian experience. Int Braz J Urol. 2021;47(6):1279–80. https://doi.org/10.1590/s1677-5538.ibju.2021.0260.
34. Kowalczyk KJ, Madi RH, Eden CG, et al. Comparative outcomes of salvage retzius-sparing versus standard robotic prostatectomy: an international, multi-surgeon series. J Urol. 2021;206(5):1184–91. https://doi.org/10.1097/JU.0000000000001939.

35. Spitznagel T, Hardenberg J, Schmid FA, et al. Salvage robotic-assisted laparoscopic radical prostatectomy following focal high-intensity focused ultrasound for ISUP 2/3 cancer. Urology. 2021;156:147–53. https://doi.org/10.1016/j.urology.2021.04.059.
36. Bozkurt Y, Atar M, Pisters LL. Early experience with salvage robotic-assisted radical prostatectomy in proton beam radiotherapy failures. Balkan Med J. 2021;38(5):310–5. https://doi.org/10.5152/balkanmedj.2021.21174.
37. Bhat KRS, Covas Moschovas M, Sandri M, et al. Outcomes of salvage robot-assisted radical prostatectomy after focal ablation for prostate cancer in comparison to primary robot-assisted radical prostatectomy: a matched analysis. Eur Urol Focus. 2022;8(5):1192–7. https://doi.org/10.1016/j.euf.2021.10.005.
38. Schuetz V, Reimold P, Goertz M, et al. Evolution of salvage radical prostatectomy from open to robotic and further to Retzius sparing surgery. J Clin Med. 2021;11(1):202. https://doi.org/10.3390/jcm11010202.
39. Blazevski A, Gondoputro W, Scheltema MJ, et al. Salvage robot-assisted radical prostatectomy following focal ablation with irreversible electroporation: feasibility, oncological and functional outcomes. BMC Urol. 2022;22(1):28. https://doi.org/10.1186/s12894-022-00978-w.
40. Mortensen MA, Poulsen CA, Ahlgren G, Madsen K, Poulsen MH. Introduction of salvage prostatectomy in Denmark: the initial experience. BMC Res Notes. 2022;15(1):185. https://doi.org/10.1186/s13104-022-06076-2.
41. Zaorsky NG, Davis BJ, Nguyen PL, et al. The evolution of brachytherapy for prostate cancer. Nat Rev Urol. 2017;14(7):415–39. https://doi.org/10.1038/nrurol.2017.76.

Technical Advances to Lymph Node Dissection: Minimizing Complications

11

Neeraja Tillu and Peter Wiklund

Abbreviations

ADC	Apparent diffusion coefficient
DW	Diffusion weighted
ePLND	extended pelvic lymph node dissection
ICG	Indocyanine green
MIS	Minimally invasive surgery
MRI	Magnetic resonance imaging
PET	Positron imaging tomography

Supplementary Information The online version contains supplementary material available at https://doi.org/10.1007/978-3-031-64245-6_11.

N. Tillu (✉)
Department of Urology, Icahn School of Medicine at Mount Sinai, New York, NY, USA
e-mail: neeraja.tillu@mountsinai.org

P. Wiklund
Department of Urology, Icahn School of Medicine at Mount Sinai, New York, NY, USA

Department of Molecular Medicine and Surgery (Solna), Karolinska Institutet, Stockholm, Sweden
e-mail: Peter.Wiklund@mountsinai.org

S. Razdan, S. Razdan (eds.), *Urinary Continence and Sexual Function After Robotic Prostatectomy, Radiation, and Novel Therapies*,
https://doi.org/10.1007/978-3-031-64245-6_11

PLND	Pelvic lymph node dissection
PPV	Positive predictive value
PSA	Prostate-specific antigen
PSMA	Prostate-specific membrane antigen
RARP	Robot-assisted radical prostatectomy
RGS	Radio-guided surgery
SNB	Sentinel node biopsy
SPECT	Single-photon emission computerized tomography
USPIO	Ultrasmall superparamagnetic iron oxide

Introduction

Pelvic lymph node dissection (PLND) is the most accurate staging for lymph node invasion in localized prostate cancer [1]. In early surgical series, lymph node metastases were noted to be as high as 40%. With increasing awareness due to prostate specific antigen (PSA) and the detection of asymptomatic prostate cancer, the reported lymph node metastases are <10% [2]. Even at this rate, the absolute number of patients with lymph node metastases remains significant. The AUA/ASTRO/SUO guideline recommends radical prostatectomy in patients with high-risk prostate cancer [3]. The therapeutic role of PLND on overall survival is unclear. However, it plays an essential role in the staging and prognostication of prostate cancer [4]. Two randomized studies have failed to show the benefit of extended PLND compared with limited [5, 6]. Current NCCN guidelines recommend the Briganti and Memorial Sloan Kettering Cancer Center (MSKCC) nomograms to predict lymph node invasion [7, 8]. These have been externally validated with comparable results [9, 10].

Limits of PLND and Short- and Long-Term Risks of PLND

PLND is the gold standard for detecting lymph node metastases in clinically localized prostate cancer [11]. Different lymph node dissection approaches have been described. Limited lymph node dissection involves obturator nodes only. Standard lymph node dissection involves the removal of the nodal tissue from between the external vein and obturator nerve, laterally from the pelvic sidewall, and the bifurcation of the iliac vessels to the femoral canal [11]. Extended PLND involves internal, external, and obturator nodes, and super-extended PLND involves internal, external, obturator, common iliac, and pre-sacral lymph nodes [12]. The risk of complications and lymph node yield increase with the extent of PLND. Extended PLND can result in threefold higher complications and a longer length of stay [13].

Lymphoceles are the most common adverse event and are associated with a greater extent of dissection. Keskin et al. noted an incidence of 9% lymphoceles in their series, of which 2.5% were symptomatic [14]. Their presentation is varied—ranging from being asymptomatic to pain, fever, lower extremity edema, and urinary and gastrointestinal problems due to mass effect on adjacent organs [15]. The surgical technique, the extent of lymph node dissection, prior radiation, and the use of heparin can contribute to an increased risk of lymphocele [16]. It is hypothesized that heparin may delay the clotting of lymphatics [17].

Other complications include deep venous thrombosis and the risk of pulmonary embolism. Munsch et al. noted that 8.3% and 2.8% of patients with lymphoceles had deep venous thrombosis and pulmonary embolism, respectively, after PLND, compared with <1% of the patients without a lymphocele [18].

Ureteric injury is another complication during PLND, and the approach does not impact the incidence of injury [15]. The obturator nerve may be injured due to clipping, transection, or thermal injury. This may require removal of the offending clip or even surgical repair, with a risk of adductor muscle impairment and loss of sensation on the medial aspect of the thigh. Gözen et al. reported a 0.1% chance of obturator nerve injury in the most extensive series of laparoscopic and robotic PLND [15]. Finally, vascular injuries are an infrequent adverse event associated with PLND, resulting in substantial blood loss and requiring swift intraoperative identification and repair [18] (Video 11.1).

Oncological Benefits of PLND

Randomized studies have shown increased lymph node yield and detectable lymph node metastases with extended and super-extended lymph node dissection compared with limited dissection [19–21]. In the randomized study by Lestingi et al., super-extended PLND had a median yield of 17 nodes compared with three nodes with limited node dissection and detected six times more nodal metastases [19]. However, no therapeutic benefit was seen from several studies, with no difference in biochemical recurrence rates and increased complications [4, 22, 23]. However, these studies are limited by selection biases in the cohort studies and limited follow-up in the clinical trials. Fossati et al. showed no benefit in biochemical recurrence, progression to distant metastases, and cancer-specific and overall survival with PLND [4]. However, they made two points that merit consideration. The authors concluded that extended lymph node dissection may provide a direct benefit by being curative in those with limited lymph node involvement [4]. It may also provide an indirect benefit by providing a stratification tool for those needing adjuvant treatment, thereby improving survival [4]. Loeb et al. reported that extended PLND may have benefits by providing biochemical recurrence in selected node-positive patients [11]. PLND has not yet demonstrated direct therapeutic benefit in prostate cancer, and further research in this area is needed.

Advances in Imaging for Lymph Node Metastases Detection

Several imaging modalities have been introduced to improve the detection of lymph node metastases during surgery using functional MR imaging and targeted PET imaging using prostate-specific membrane antigen (PSMA). Ultrasmall superparamagnetic iron oxide (USPIO)-enhanced MR imaging, diffusion-weighted (DW) MR imaging, and a combination of these two methods have increased the accuracy of lymph node detection using MRI [24]. In the proPSMA study, the authors found a lower sensitivity (38% vs 85%) and specificity (91% vs 98%) for bone scan and CT compared with PSMA PET-CT [25].

1. USPIO-enhanced MRI imaging has been extensively studied in detecting lymph node metastases. In a prospective study, MRI using Ferumoxtran-10 correctly identified all patients with lymph node metastases and had higher sensitivity than conventional MRI (90.5% vs 35.4%, $P < 0.001$) [26]. In another study using USPIO-enhanced MRI in bladder and prostate cancer, the first reading had a sensitivity of 55.0% and diagnostic accuracy of 77.3%. The second reading had a mean sensitivity of 58.3% and an accuracy of 76.4%. Most missed metastases were smaller than 5 mm in diameter [27]. However, several challenges exist in the administration of ferumoxtran, including unavailability, infusion reactions, and missing metastases <5 mm. Ferumoxytol is similar in concept to Ferumoxtran-10 and addresses some of its limitations. However, extensive studies have yet to prove that ferumoxytol produces results comparable with ferumoxtran-10.
2. DW imaging depicts how much the tissue structure impedes the Brownian motion of water molecules. Lymph nodes harboring malignancy will have impeded diffusion and lower apparent diffusion coefficient (ADC) values. Although ADC can differentiate between benign and malignant, it has sensitivities and specificities ranging from 76.4% to 100% and 74% to 98.3%, respectively [28]. Alternatively, MR imaging with a high b-value can be used as normal tissue does not retain signal, whereas malignant nodes retain signal, thereby creating high contrast T2 images. This has sensitivities ranging from 75.8% to 81.8% and specificity of 95.4% [24]. It is widely available and nonquantitative and does not require a contrast agent. However, it can be inaccurate while reporting small nodes as the images can be noisy and need correlation with morphological images to avoid mistaking vascular structures and nerves for lymph nodes.
3. Combination of USPIO and DW imaging

   This can improve lymph node imaging further as benign LNs are not visible on DW images, and malignant LNs remain hyperintense with high b-values due to the lack of contrast uptake [29]. In a study of 75 patients, the combination of USPIO had sensitivity and specificity ranges of 65–75% and 93–96%, respectively. However, these studies remain limited by a small number of patients.
4. Functional Imaging: Positron emission tomography (PET) using tracers such as fluorodeoxyglucose and choline has gained limited traction over recent years as these are not helpful in the setting of biochemical recurrence or early metastatic

disease [30, 31]. Prostate-specific membrane antigen (PSMA) is a transmembrane glycoprotein overexpressed in prostate cancer cells [30]. Gallium 68 (68Ga) or Fluorine 18 (18F) radiolabeled PSMA ligands are currently in use for the primary staging of prostate cancer [16]. These have greater sensitivity and specificity than choline PET scans due to higher tumor-to-background contrast. The most widely studied is 68Ga-PSMA PET/CT scan. In a meta-analysis by Perera et al. involving five studies, the sensitivity and specificity of PSMA PET scan were 77% and 97%, respectively, on a per-patient analysis [30]. In a retrospective study from Sweden, the sensitivity and specificity of [18F] PSMA-1007 in high- and intermediate-risk PCa to detect a lymph node metastasis $\geq$3 mm on PET/CT were 53.8% and 96.7%, respectively [32]. The current evidence suggests that 68Ga PSMA PET/CT scan shows excellent promise in the primary lymph node staging of PCa due to its high sensitivity and PPV. Further studies are required before using PSMA PET scan as the standard of care in high- and intermediate-risk prostate cancer in replacing extended pelvic lymph node dissection (ePLND).

Sentinel Lymph Node Biopsy for PLND

Sentinel node biopsy (SNB) analysis is based on the criteria that sentinel nodes are the first to be involved in migrating tumor cells. Various ^{99m}Tc-labeled colloids and ultrasmall super magnetic nanoparticle MRI have been used as radiotracers [33]. Radiotracers and indocyanine green (ICG) are administered into the prostate under transrectal or transperineal guidance [34]. Preoperatively, lymphoscintigraphy or SPECT-CT are used to detect the sentinel nodes, with improved detection in the latter [35]. Intraoperatively, a gamma-ray detection probe, gamma camera, navigation systems with freehand SPECT technology, or a fluorescence camera help detect hotspots or fluorescence depending on the technology used [33]. A systematic review did not show any benefit of SNB over ePLND, although it appears to increase the nodal yield when combined with ePLND [36]. There is insufficient evidence to support SNB in PLND at present.

Advances in Surgical Techniques for Lymph Node Dissection

With time, pelvic lymph node dissection has progressed from open to laparoscopic and robotic. The minimally invasive techniques have the advantage of less blood loss, shortened length of stay, and decreased postoperative pain [37]. Patients with locally advanced disease were traditionally considered for systemic therapy upfront [38]. However, recent studies demonstrate that surgery in combination with androgen deprivation therapy and radiotherapy is an oncologically safe option in locally advanced disease [39]. Mottrie et al. studied robot-assisted radical prostatectomy (RARP) with ePLND in patients with locally advanced diseases in three high-volume European centers and found excellent perioperative results and long-term follow-up [40]. Two out of three patients were recurrence-free at 3 years follow-up. They observed that RARP in the hands of experienced surgeons caused reduced blood loss, improved magnification, and three-dimensional vision, which led to better cancer control.

Lymphoceles are the most common complication after PLND and can lead to substantial morbidity. Monopolar or bipolar coagulation of lymphatic vessels has shown poor sealing of lymphatic vessels compared with clipping in one study [41]. In another prospective study, no difference has been shown between bipolar coagulation and titanium clipping for lymphatic vessels [42]. These methods are controversial. Other strategies to control lymphatic leak include fibrin glue [43] and the use of hemostatic patches [44], whose benefits are not yet proven. Yasumizu et al. showed that vessel sealing devices (EnSeal®, Ethicon Inc., Cincinnati, USA) can prevent formation of lymphoceles [45]. Abaza et al. found that robotic vessel sealer did not increase lymphoceles compared with clips [46]. Recently published studies have established that peritoneal flap or peritoneal fenestration can decrease symptomatic and asymptomatic lymphoceles due to increased resorption [47].

PSMA-Guided Radiosurgery

PSMA-guided radiosurgery (RGS) has been studied as a method to guide lymph node dissection and defer systemic therapy [48]. Results from the DETECT study confirmed the feasibility of PSMA-guided radiosurgery in 12 patients [49]. In a study by Lunger et al., PSMA-guided radiosurgery facilitated the detection of lymph nodes in 94% of patients [50]. In the study by Knipper et al., 99mTc-PSMA-I&S or 111In-PSMA-I&T is prepared and injected intravenously the day prior to surgery [48]. CT is performed one day prior to surgery to cross-validate the PSMA PET findings and find the dominant lesion. A gamma probe is used intraoperatively to measure the radioactivity of PSMA tracers. This is helpful in salvage PLNDs with fibrosis at the site of surgery. Ex vivo gamma measurements confirm the removal of nodes and prompt further search if there is a missing signal. PSMA RGS remains experimental, and randomized prospective data are needed before its incorporation in clinical practice.

Conclusion

PLND is an indicated procedure for high-risk prostate cancer patients. The extent of dissection needs to be calculated for each patient and is associated with complications, but the oncological benefit remains controversial. Continued refinements in surgical technique coupled with patient selection can reduce morbidity. SNB and imaging have advanced to detect lymph nodes, and PSMA PET scan shows great promise due to its high specificity and positive predictive value. Advances in minimally invasive surgery (MIS) and PSMA-guided surgery are other technical advancements that help minimize complications of PLND. Further high-quality level 1 evidence is needed for its routine use in daily practice.

Take-Home Message

The debate still continues on whether PLND improves oncological outcomes in men with prostate cancer. While there is some data on its utility in treating regional lymph node metastasis, most PLND is performed for its prognostication ability and accurate staging. To minimize the adverse events associated with PLND, surgeons must take care to avoid damage to nearby neural and vascular structures. The use of clips and thermal energy can also be used to prevent lymphocele formation, which while often asymptomatic, can manifest with irritative voiding symptoms postoperatively due to extrinsic compression of the bladder.

References

1. Aus G, Abbou CC, Bolla M, et al. EAU guidelines on prostate cancer. Eur Urol. 2005;48:546–51. https://doi.org/10.1016/j.eururo.2005.06.001.
2. Swanson GP, Thompson IM, Basler J. Current status of lymph node-positive prostate cancer. Cancer. 2006;107:439–50. https://doi.org/10.1002/cncr.22034.
3. Eastham JA, Auffenberg GB, Barocas DA, et al. Clinically localized prostate cancer: AUA/ASTRO guideline, part I: introduction, risk assessment, staging, and risk-based management. J Urol. 2022;208:10–8. https://doi.org/10.1097/JU.0000000000002757.
4. Fossati N, Willemse P-PM, Van den Broeck T, et al. The benefits and harms of different extents of lymph node dissection during radical prostatectomy for prostate cancer: a systematic review. Eur Urol. 2017;72:84–109. https://doi.org/10.1016/j.eururo.2016.12.003.
5. Lestingi JFP, Guglielmetti GB, Trinh Q-D, et al. Extended versus limited pelvic lymph node dissection during radical prostatectomy for intermediate- and high-risk prostate cancer: early oncological outcomes from a randomized phase 3 trial. Eur Urol. 2021;79:595–604. https://doi.org/10.1016/j.eururo.2020.11.040.
6. Touijer KA, Sjoberg DD, Benfante N, et al. Limited versus extended pelvic lymph node dissection for prostate cancer: a randomized clinical trial. Eur Urol Oncol. 2021;4:532–9. https://doi.org/10.1016/j.euo.2021.03.006.
7. Gandaglia G, Fossati N, Zaffuto E, et al. Development and internal validation of a novel model to identify the candidates for extended pelvic lymph node dissection in prostate cancer. Eur Urol. 2017;72:632–40. https://doi.org/10.1016/j.eururo.2017.03.049.
8. www.mskcc.org/nomograms/prostate/pre_op
9. Hueting TA, Cornel EB, Somford DM, et al. External validation of models predicting the probability of lymph node involvement in prostate cancer patients. Eur Urol Oncol. 2018;1:411–7. https://doi.org/10.1016/j.euo.2018.04.016.
10. Hansen J, Rink M, Bianchi M, et al. External validation of the updated briganti nomogram to predict lymph node invasion in prostate cancer patients undergoing extended lymph node dissection. Prostate. 2013;73:211–8. https://doi.org/10.1002/pros.22559.
11. Loeb S, Partin AW, Schaeffer EM. Complications of pelvic lymphadenectomy: do the risks outweigh the benefits? Rev Urol. 2010;12:20–4.
12. Mattei A, Fuechsel FG, Bhatta Dhar N, et al. The template of the primary lymphatic landing sites of the prostate should be revisited: results of a multimodality mapping study. Eur Urol. 2008;53:118–25. https://doi.org/10.1016/j.eururo.2007.07.035.

13. Briganti A, Chun FK-H, Salonia A, et al. Complications and other surgical outcomes associated with extended pelvic lymphadenectomy in men with localized prostate cancer. Eur Urol. 2006;50:1006–13. https://doi.org/10.1016/j.eururo.2006.08.015.
14. Keskin MS, Argun ÖB, Öbek C, et al. The incidence and sequela of lymphocele formation after robot-assisted extended pelvic lymph node dissection. BJU Int. 2016;118:127–31. https://doi.org/10.1111/bju.13425.
15. Keegan KA, Cookson MS. Complications of pelvic lymph node dissection for prostate cancer. Curr Urol Rep. 2011;12:203–8. https://doi.org/10.1007/s11934-011-0179-z.
16. Haxhimolla J, Kua B, Gilbourd D, Haxhimolla H. PSMA PET scan era: a changing paradigm PSMA PET and lymph node dissection for prostate cancer management. Semin Oncol Nurs. 2020;36:151044. https://doi.org/10.1016/j.soncn.2020.151044.
17. Catalona WJ, Kadmon D, Crane DB. Effect of mini-dose heparin on lymphocele formation following extraperitoneal pelvic lymphadenectomy. J Urol. 1980;123:890–2. https://doi.org/10.1016/S0022-5347(17)56180-7.
18. Musch M, Klevecka V, Roggenbuck U, Kroepfl D. Complications of pelvic lymphadenectomy in 1,380 patients undergoing radical retropubic prostatectomy between 1993 and 2006. J Urol. 2008;179:923–9. https://doi.org/10.1016/j.juro.2007.10.072.
19. Lestingi JFP, Guglielmetti G, Pontes J Jr, et al. Extended versus limited pelvic lymphadenectomy during radical prostatectomy for intermediate- and high-risk prostate cancer: early outcomes from a randomized controlled phase III study. J Clin Oncol. 2017;35:5018. https://doi.org/10.1200/JCO.2017.35.15_suppl.5018.
20. Schwerfeld-Bohr J, Kaemper M, Krege S, Heidenreich A. 270 prospective randomized multicenter study comparing limited vs extended pelvic lymphadenectomy in intermediate and high risk prostate cancer—comparison of complications (SEAL, AUO AP 55/09). Eur Urol Suppl. 2014;13:e270. https://doi.org/10.1016/S1569-9056(14)60266-9.
21. Clark T, Parekh DJ, Cookson MS, et al. Randomized prospective evaluation of extended versus limited lymph node dissection in patients with clinically localized prostate cancer. J Urol. 2003;169:145–8. https://doi.org/10.1016/S0022-5347(05)64055-4.
22. Chen J, Wang Z, Zhao J, et al. Pelvic lymph node dissection and its extent on survival benefit in prostate cancer patients with a risk of lymph node invasion >5%: a propensity score matching analysis from SEER database. Sci Rep. 2019;9:17985. https://doi.org/10.1038/s41598-019-54261-4.
23. Preisser F, van den Bergh RCN, Gandaglia G, et al. Effect of extended pelvic lymph node dissection on oncologic outcomes in patients with D'Amico intermediate and high risk prostate cancer treated with radical prostatectomy: a multi-institutional study. J Urol. 2020;203:338–43. https://doi.org/10.1097/JU.0000000000000504.
24. Thoeny HC, Barbieri S, Froehlich JM, et al. Functional and targeted lymph node imaging in prostate cancer: current status and future challenges. Radiology. 2017;285:728–43. https://doi.org/10.1148/radiol.2017161517.
25. Hofman MS, Lawrentschuk N, Francis RJ, et al. Prostate-specific membrane antigen PET-CT in patients with high-risk prostate cancer before curative-intent surgery or radiotherapy (proPSMA): a prospective, randomised, multicentre study. Lancet. 2020;395:1208–16. https://doi.org/10.1016/S0140-6736(20)30314-7.
26. Harisinghani MG, Barentsz J, Hahn PF, et al. Noninvasive detection of clinically occult lymph-node metastases in prostate cancer. N Engl J Med. 2003;348:2491–9. https://doi.org/10.1056/NEJMoa022749.
27. Triantafyllou M, Studer UE, Birkhäuser FD, et al. Ultrasmall superparamagnetic particles of iron oxide allow for the detection of metastases in normal sized pelvic lymph nodes of patients with bladder and/or prostate cancer. Eur J Cancer. 2013;49:616–24. https://doi.org/10.1016/j.ejca.2012.09.034.
28. Park SY, Oh YT, Jung DC, et al. Prediction of micrometastasis (<1 cm) to pelvic lymph nodes in prostate cancer: role of preoperative MRI. Am J Roentgenol. 2015;205:W328–34. https://doi.org/10.2214/AJR.14.14138.

29. Birkhäuser FD, Studer UE, Froehlich JM, et al. Combined ultrasmall superparamagnetic particles of iron oxide–enhanced and diffusion-weighted magnetic resonance imaging facilitates detection of metastases in normal-sized pelvic lymph nodes of patients with bladder and prostate cancer. Eur Urol. 2013;64:953–60. https://doi.org/10.1016/j.eururo.2013.07.032.
30. Perera M, Papa N, Roberts M, et al. Gallium-68 prostate-specific membrane antigen positron emission tomography in advanced prostate cancer—updated diagnostic utility, sensitivity, specificity, and distribution of prostate-specific membrane antigen-avid lesions: a systematic review and meta-analysis. Eur Urol. 2020;77:403–17. https://doi.org/10.1016/j.eururo.2019.01.049.
31. Eapen RS, Nzenza TC, Murphy DG, et al. PSMA PET applications in the prostate cancer journey: from diagnosis to theranostics. World J Urol. 2019;37:1255–61. https://doi.org/10.1007/s00345-018-2524-z.
32. Ingvar J, Hvittfeldt E, Trägårdh E, et al. Assessing the accuracy of [18F]PSMA-1007 PET/CT for primary staging of lymph node metastases in intermediate- and high-risk prostate cancer patients. EJNMMI Res. 2022;12:48. https://doi.org/10.1186/s13550-022-00918-7.
33. Acar C, Kleinjan GH, van den Berg NS, et al. Advances in sentinel node dissection in prostate cancer from a technical perspective. Int J Urol. 2015;22:898–909. https://doi.org/10.1111/iju.12863.
34. Jeschke S, Lusuardi L, Myatt A, et al. Visualisation of the lymph node pathway in real time by laparoscopic radioisotope- and fluorescence-guided sentinel lymph node dissection in prostate cancer staging. Urology. 2012;80:1080–7. https://doi.org/10.1016/j.urology.2012.05.050.
35. Warncke SH, Mattei A, Fuechsel FG, et al. Detection rate and operating time required for γ probe-guided sentinel lymph node resection after injection of technetium-99m nanocolloid into the prostate with and without preoperative imaging. Eur Urol. 2007;52:126–33. https://doi.org/10.1016/j.eururo.2007.01.050.
36. Wit EMK, Acar C, Grivas N, et al. Sentinel node procedure in prostate cancer: a systematic review to assess diagnostic accuracy. Eur Urol. 2017;71:596–605. https://doi.org/10.1016/j.eururo.2016.09.007.
37. Guillonneau B, Cathelineau X, Doublet J-D, et al. Laparoscopic radical prostatectomy: assessment after 550 procedures. Crit Rev Oncol Hematol. 2002;43:123–33. https://doi.org/10.1016/S1040-8428(02)00024-0.
38. Lowrance WT, Elkin EB, Yee DS, et al. Locally advanced prostate cancer: a population-based study of treatment patterns. BJU Int. 2012;109:1309–14. https://doi.org/10.1111/j.1464-410X.2011.10760.x.
39. Gözen AS, Akin Y, Ates M, et al. Impact of laparoscopic radical prostatectomy on clinical T3 prostate cancer: experience of a single centre with long-term follow-up. BJU Int. 2015;116:102–8. https://doi.org/10.1111/bju.12710.
40. Gandaglia G, De Lorenzis E, Novara G, et al. Robot-assisted radical prostatectomy and extended pelvic lymph node dissection in patients with locally-advanced prostate cancer. Eur Urol. 2017;71:249–56. https://doi.org/10.1016/j.eururo.2016.05.008.
41. Porter K, O'Connor S, Rimm E, Lopez M. Electrocautery as a factor in seroma formation following mastectomy. Am J Surg. 1998;176:8–11. https://doi.org/10.1016/S0002-9610(98)00093-2.
42. Grande P, Di Pierro GB, Mordasini L, et al. Prospective randomized trial comparing titanium clips to bipolar coagulation in sealing lymphatic vessels during pelvic lymph node dissection at the time of robot-assisted radical prostatectomy. Eur Urol. 2017;71:155–8. https://doi.org/10.1016/j.eururo.2016.08.006.
43. Garayev A, Aytaç Ö, Tavukcu HH, Atug F. Effect of autologous fibrin glue on lymphatic drainage and lymphocele formation in extended bilateral pelvic lymphadenectomy in robot-assisted radical prostatectomy. J Endourol. 2019;33:761–6. https://doi.org/10.1089/end.2018.0853.
44. Buelens S, Van Praet C, Poelaert F, et al. Prospective randomized controlled trial exploring the effect of TachoSil on lymphocele formation after extended pelvic lymph node dissection in prostate cancer. Urology. 2018;118:134–40. https://doi.org/10.1016/j.urology.2018.05.008.

45. Yasumizu Y, Miyajima A, Maeda T, et al. How can lymphocele development be prevented after laparoscopic radical prostatectomy? J Endourol. 2013;27:447–51. https://doi.org/10.1089/end.2012.0356.
46. Abaza R, Henderson SJ, Martinez O. Robotic vessel sealer device for lymphocele prevention after pelvic lymphadenectomy: results of a randomized trial. J Laparoendosc Adv Surg Tech. 2022;32:721–6. https://doi.org/10.1089/lap.2021.0531.
47. Lebeis C, Canes D, Sorcini A, Moinzadeh A. Novel technique prevents lymphoceles after transperitoneal robotic-assisted pelvic lymph node dissection: peritoneal flap interposition. Urology. 2015;85:1505–9. https://doi.org/10.1016/j.urology.2015.02.034.
48. Knipper S, Mehdi Irai M, Simon R, et al. Cohort study of Oligorecurrent prostate cancer patients: oncological outcomes of patients treated with salvage lymph node dissection via prostate-specific membrane antigen–radioguided surgery. Eur Urol. 2023;83:62–9. https://doi.org/10.1016/j.eururo.2022.05.031.
49. Gondoputro W, Scheltema MJ, Blazevski A, et al. Robot-assisted prostate-specific membrane antigen-radioguided surgery in primary diagnosed prostate cancer. J Nucl Med. 2022;jnumed.121.263743:jnumed.121.263743. https://doi.org/10.2967/jnumed.121.263743.
50. Lunger L, Steinhelfer L, Korn P, et al. Prostate-specific membrane antigen–radioguided surgery facilitates pelvic lymph node dissection during radical prostatectomy for the treatment of locally advanced prostate cancer with regional lymph node metastases. Eur Urol Oncol. 2023;6:95–8. https://doi.org/10.1016/j.euo.2022.12.001.

Functional Outcomes of Prostate Cancer Treatment with Partial Gland Ablation

12

Basil Kaufmann, Dallin Busby, and Michael A. Gorin

Introduction

The widespread use of PSA testing has resulted in a significant increase in the detection of early-stage prostate cancer [1, 2]. While active surveillance remains the preferred management strategy for men with grade group 1 prostate cancer, individuals with grade group ≥2 disease typically require treatment with either radical prostatectomy or radiation therapy. Although these whole gland treatment strategies offer high efficacy in terms of cancer control, their use is associated with unacceptably high risk of quality of life alternating functional declines in erectile and urinary function. For example, Haglind et al. [3] reported in a prospective randomized controlled trial of robotic versus open prostatectomy that 20% of men were found to have urinary incontinence requiring at least one pad per 24 hours at 12 months regardless of the surgical technique used. In addition, 70% of men had permanent erectile dysfunction (ED). After radiation therapy, 3% of patients reported no control or frequent urinary leakage, while ED was reported by 60% at 2 years and 70% of patients at 5 years [4]. As a result, there has been considerable interest in the development of partial gland treatments that allow for the avoidance of collateral damage to the neurovascular bundles and continence mechanism.

A growing body of evidence exists in support of the use of subtotal ablative techniques for the treatment of prostate cancer. However, it is important to note that the

B. Kaufmann (✉)
Milton and Carroll Petrie Department of Urology, Icahn School of Medicine at Mount Sinai, New York, NY, USA

Department of Urology, University Hospital Zurich, Zurich, Switzerland

D. Busby · M. A. Gorin
Milton and Carroll Petrie Department of Urology, Icahn School of Medicine at Mount Sinai, New York, NY, USA
e-mail: dallin.busby@mountsinai.org; michael.gorin@mountsinai.org

S. Razdan, S. Razdan (eds.), *Urinary Continence and Sexual Function After Robotic Prostatectomy, Radiation, and Novel Therapies*,
https://doi.org/10.1007/978-3-031-64245-6_12

majority of available data on prostate cancer ablation comes from non-comparative, single center, and/or retrospective studies. In addition, heterogeneity exists in the techniques used as well as the way functional and oncologic outcomes are defined. As a result, current guidelines do not yet support the routine use of subtotal ablative approaches for the treatment of prostate cancer. Nonetheless, this treatment approach continues to be used clinically. In this chapter, we outline the potential functional benefits of subtotal prostate ablation for the treatment of prostate cancer, while acknowledging the limitations of the available literature on this topic.

Principles of Subtotal Prostate Ablation

The anatomy of the prostate and surrounding structures has important implications for subtotal or partial gland ablation. The neurovascular bundles, which contain the cavernous nerves that are critical for erectile function, run along the posterolateral border of the prostate. The smooth muscle that runs from the bladder neck through the prostate to the membranous urethra provides passive continence, while the outer rhabdo sphincter maintains the active continence. Fibers of the rhabdosphincter extend anteriorly and blend with prostate tissue near the apex. The prostate borders the pubic symphysis anteriorly and the rectum posteriorly, separated only by a thin fascial layer called Denonvilliers fascia [5].

Given this anatomy, treatments for prostate cancer that involve even only ablating a part of the gland may put the neurovascular bundles, sphincter, and rectum at risk for damage. As a general rule, the more prostate tissue ablated, the higher the risk of impairment to erectile function, urinary continence, and rectal injury. As we know from the practice of radical prostatectomy, great care in the apex is needed, to maintain the integrity of both muscular sphincteric parts [6]. Therefore, the apical anatomy and the close proximity to the external sphincter require careful treatment planning at the time of prostate ablation [7]. Considering the rectum's close proximity posteriorly, vigilance is required at the time of ablation to prevent injury to this structure. The risk of developing a recto-urethral fistula is increased when treatment is performed in a salvage setting or when the cancer is located in the prostate's posterior region [8].

While the targeted focal approach seeks to maintain the best functional outcomes, it may be viewed as a potential compromise from an oncological standpoint. Given that prostate cancer is a multifocal disease with approximately 80% of cases containing multiple foci [9], concerns persist regarding oncologic outcomes using partial gland ablation. However, it should be noted that available long-term outcomes in terms of metastasis-free survival, progression-free survival, and cancer-specific survival appear to be very promising. Oncological outcomes of focal HIFU in Europe have reported rates of absence of clinically significant disease in follow-up biopsies of 81% [10] at 12 months and 73% at 30 months [11] post-treatment. Furthermore, freedom from radical or systemic therapy, metastases, and cancer-specific mortality were 99% at 1 year, 92% at 3 years, and 88% at 5 years [12]. Cryotherapy, on the other hand, has demonstrated cancer-specific and metastasis-free survival of 100% at 3–5 years [13–15] and a 10-year systemic treatment-free rate of 65% [16].

Impact on Erectile Function

Fiard et al. [17] conducted a recent systematic review and meta-analysis that focused on the impact of partial gland ablation on sexual outcomes using patient-reported outcome questionnaires. The study included 42 studies with a total of 2367 patients, of which 50% had baseline self-reported potency scores available, comprising 1317 patients. The preoperative potency scores were defined by each study and 70% of the patients were found to be potent with erections sufficient for penetration. HIFU was the most commonly used energy source, applied in 45% of the cases, followed by cryotherapy in 21%. Targeted photodynamic therapy and irreversible electroporation were the least studied techniques, with 7% and 8%, respectively. Hemiablation (n = 953) and targeted focal ablation (n = 1039) were the most frequently used treatment templates. Across all treatment types and ablation patterns, the authors found a decrease in early sexual function after partial gland ablation at 3 months postoperatively (−3.70 [95% CI −4.43 to −2.96] change in IIEF-5 score), with relative improvement at 6 months (−2.18 [−2.91 to −1.46]) and 12 months (−2.14 [−2.96 to −1.32]) [17]. No statistically significant difference was found between the different types of energy at 6 and 12 months ($p = 0.36$ and 0.69, respectively). However, the worst outcomes were observed in a study using a hockey-stick cryoablation template, with a 3- and 6-month outcome of −12.80 and −11.95, respectively [18].

When interpreting these results, it is important to consider that there is a lack of consensus on the most appropriate outcome measures to use for assessing post-treatment sexual function after prostate ablation. As a result, studies have reported results in a variety of ways, with most focusing on either a binary determination of potency or changes in survey scores. In addition, most studies do not take into account confounding factors such as baseline potency or treatment with PDE5 inhibitors. Furthermore, the IIEF-5 questionnaire that was mostly used was originally designed and validated for men with ED in stable relationships with female partners for at least 6 months, while its use among sexual minorities and its measurement properties have been questioned [19, 20]. In addition, the questionnaire only focuses on erectile function and does not consider other aspects of sexual function such as orgasmic or ejaculatory function, sexual desire, or masculinity/virility issues. Furthermore, dropout rates are high, with up to 76% of patients not completing all post-operative questionnaires [17].

The comparison of ED rates between whole gland treatments (i.e., radical prostatectomy, radiotherapy, or brachytherapy) and partial gland ablation indicates more favorable outcomes for the latter [21]. A prospective multicenter study looked at 1027 men who underwent whole gland treatment [22]. Two years post-treatment, 65% of men in the radical prostatectomy group, 63% in the radiotherapy group, and 57% in the brachytherapy group reported ED. Furthermore, in ProtecT trial [23], only 18% of the prostatectomy group reported erections sufficient for sexual intercourse at 7 years.

Ejaculation dysfunction is another significant side effect of whole gland treatments for many men. Although a "dry orgasm" after radical prostatectomy is possible, some patients have reported a reduction in the intensity or enjoyment of their orgasms [24]. However, this may also be attributed to psychological factors rather than the radical prostatectomy procedure itself [25]. In partial gland ablation, ejaculation dysfunction seems to be uncommon. Three prospective studies on HIFU reported ejaculation-related adverse events [26–28]. Ganzer et al. [26] observed one patient out of 51 experiencing anejaculation, while one suffered pain during ejaculation. Hardenberg et al. [27] found one out of 24 patients with anejaculation, and Shoji et al. [28] reported that 70% of patients were still able to maintain ejaculation 12 months after treatment. Two phase 2 trials [29] on vascular targeted photodynamic therapy reported over a 3.5-year period that 5 out of 68 patients reported Clavien Dindo grade I ejaculation sequelae. Based on these findings, it appears that partial gland ablation using HIFU and vascular targeted photodynamic therapy may mostly preserve ejaculation function while further research is needed [21].

Impact on Urinary Continence

Much of the literature on urinary incontinence after partial gland ablation is based on single center or retrospective studies and is generally considered to be low quality. With that said, a recent meta-analysis by Hopstaken et al. [30] has reported aggregate results. The review analyzed 72 studies that applied eight different sources of energy. The assessment of urinary incontinence varied across studies, with most reporting either "pad-free" or "leak-free" rates without implementing established questionnaire scores. The review found that after HIFU, a median of 95% of patients were pad-free after a follow-up ≥1 year, including patients after transurethral resection of the prostate ($n = 10$) and without ($n = 17$). Irreversible electroporation studies ($n = 9$) and focal laser ablation studies ($n = 8$) showed a median of 100% pad-free patients after treatment. Focal cryoablation studies reported 100% pad-free continence in four out of five studies that reported on continence changes. Two studies have compared focal cryoablation with whole gland cryoablation. One study found no significant difference in pad-free continence between the two groups (both 83%) [31]. The other study reported a significant difference in favor of focal cryotherapy, with a 100% pad-free continence rate at 24 months compared to 98.7% for whole gland cryoablation ($p = 0.02$) [32]. Photodynamic therapy ($n = 7$) and focal brachytherapy studies ($n = 8$) did not report any changes in continence. Radiofrequency ablation ($n = 2$) studies reported no pad use in one study [33], while the other reported that 2 out of 18 patients required a pad after treatment [34].

Compared to other treatments for localized prostate cancer, partial gland ablation has demonstrated superior urinary continence rates. For example, in the ProtecT trial, [23] patients who underwent prostatectomy experienced urinary leakage requiring pads in 18 to 24% of cases, whereas the active monitoring group and radiotherapy group experienced rates of 9–11% and 3–8%, respectively. Radiotherapy may also induce irritative lower urinary tract symptoms immediately after therapy, while many patients requiring alphablockers [35, 36].

Recovery of incontinence after partial gland ablation will occur naturally in most of the cases, but some patients may require pelvic floor physiotherapy. There is no evidence or case studies indicating the necessity of artificial urinary sphincter or other invasive procedures after partial gland ablation for prostate cancer [8].

Limitations of the Present Literature

Although partial gland ablation aims to lead to improved functional outcomes for men with prostate cancer, measuring and comparing functional outcomes presents a challenging task due to several factors. Firstly, the use of different forms of energies and treatment templates can lead to variations in outcomes. Very few head-to-head studies compare outcomes for different energy sources. It is, therefore, difficult to ascertain the degree to which outcomes for one particular energy source are generalizable to other energy sources. Secondly, many studies are still in the early research stages, which mean that there is a learning curve involved in either the surgical technique or the selection and extent of treatment. Moreover, follow-up protocols differ from one study to another, adding to the complexity of comparing outcomes. Lastly, it is important to note that certain outcomes reported by physicians may not accurately reflect the patient's perspective [30]. This discrepancy was highlighted in the patient-led EUPROMS study [37], which found that physician-reported outcome measures may not accurately reflect what patients consider to be a positive outcome. Despite these challenges, systematic reviews help us in consolidating the existing evidence, evaluating the quality and potential bias of the studies, and identifying areas for further research.

Conclusion

Based on the current literature, the risk of new onset ED after partial gland ablation is notably lower than that following whole gland treatments, while the incidence of urinary incontinence appears to be rare. Regardless of the energy source applied, pad-free continence rates range from 95% to 100%, while leak-free continence rates range from 83% to 100%. In terms of ED, most patients will experience a decline in the initial 3 months following treatment, but the majority will recover function close to their baseline level thereafter. When considering these functional benefits, it is important to weigh the potential concerns of oncologic control which is typically inferior to the outcomes of whole gland treatments. With that said, given the long natural history of prostate cancer and the many options for salvage treatment, this so far does not appear to translate to increased risk of prostate cancer-related death.

Take-Home Message

Focal therapy and partial gland ablation are increasingly sought after treatments by patients due to their reduced risk of urinary and erectile side effects. Long-term disease specific survival is predicated on accurate targeting of suspicious lesions with the use of pre-procedural mpMRI to ensure complete destruction of malignant tissue.

References

1. Cooperberg MR, Broering JM, Kantoff PW, et al. Contemporary trends in low risk prostate cancer: risk assessment and treatment. J Urol. 2007;178:S14.
2. Fletcher SA, Von Landenberg N, Cole AP, et al. Contemporary national trends in prostate cancer risk profile at diagnosis. Prostate Cancer Prostatic Dis. 2020;23:81.
3. Haglind E, Carlsson S, Stranne J, et al. Urinary incontinence and erectile dysfunction after robotic versus open radical prostatectomy: a prospective, controlled, nonrandomised trial. Eur Urol. 2015;68:216.
4. Resnick MJ, Koyama T, Fan K-H, et al. Long-term functional outcomes after treatment for localized prostate cancer. N Engl J Med. 2013;368:436.
5. Costello AJ, Corcoran NM. Development, applied, and surgical anatomy of the prostate. In: Tewari A, editor. Prostate cancer: a comprehensive perspective. London: Springer; 2013. p. 3–17.
6. Myers RP, Goellner JR, Cahill DR. Prostate shape, external striated urethral sphincter and radical prostatectomy: the apical dissection. J Urol. 1987;138:543.
7. Villers A, Tay KJ. Focal therapy for anterior cancers (originated from transition zone). In: Polascik T, editor. Imaging and focal therapy of early prostate cancer. Cham: Springer; 2017. p. 373.
8. Rakauskas A, Marra G, Heidegger I, et al. Focal therapy for prostate cancer: complications and their treatment. Front Surg. 2021;8:696242.
9. Karavitakis M, Ahmed HU, Abel PD, et al. Tumor focality in prostate cancer: implications for focal therapy. Nat Rev Clin Oncol. 2011;8:48.
10. Ahmed HU, Dickinson L, Charman S, et al. Focal ablation targeted to the index lesion in multifocal localised prostate cancer: a prospective development study. Eur Urol. 2015;68:927.
11. Johnston MJ, Emara A, Noureldin M, et al. Focal high-intensity focussed ultrasound partial gland ablation for the treatment of localised prostate cancer: a report of medium-term outcomes from a single-center in the United Kingdom. Urology. 2019;133:175.
12. Guillaumier S, Peters M, Arya M, et al. A multicentre study of 5-year outcomes following focal therapy in treating clinically significant nonmetastatic prostate cancer. Eur Urol. 2018;74:422.
13. Shah TT, Peters M, Eldred-Evans D, et al. Early-medium-term outcomes of primary focal cryotherapy to treat nonmetastatic clinically significant prostate cancer from a prospective multicentre registry. Eur Urol. 2019;76:98.
14. Oishi M, Gill IS, Tafuri A, et al. Hemigland cryoablation of localized low, intermediate and high risk prostate cancer: oncologic and functional outcomes at 5 years. J Urol. 2019;202:1188.
15. Tan WP, Chang A, Sze C, et al. Oncological and functional outcomes of patients undergoing individualized partial gland cryoablation of the prostate: a single-institution experience. J Endourol. 2021;35:1290.
16. Marra G, Soeterik T, Oreggia D, et al. Long-term outcomes of focal cryotherapy for low- to intermediate-risk prostate cancer: results and matched pair analysis with active surveillance. Eur Urol Focus. 2022;8:701.
17. Fiard G, Chowdhury A, Potter AR, et al. Detailing sexual outcomes after focal therapy for localised prostate cancer: a systematic review and meta-analysis. Eur Urol Focus. 2022;8:926.

18. Gregg JR, Borregales LD, Choi H, et al. Prospective trial of regional (hockey-stick) prostate cryoablation: oncologic and quality of life outcomes. World J Urol. 2021;39:3259.
19. Rosen RC, Allen KR, Ni X, et al. Minimal clinically important differences in the erectile function domain of the international index of erectile function scale. Eur Urol. 2011;60:1010.
20. Neijenhuijs KI, Holtmaat K, Aaronson NK, et al. The international index of erectile function (IIEF)—a systematic review of measurement properties. J Sex Med. 2019;16:1078.
21. Ramacciotti LS, Jadvar DS, Lenon MSL, et al. Focal therapy for prostate cancer: the impact on sexual function. Uro. 2022;2:204.
22. Alemozaffar M, Regan MM, Cooperberg MR, et al. Prediction of erectile function following treatment for prostate cancer. JAMA. 2011;306:1205.
23. Donovan JL, Hamdy FC, Lane JA, et al. Patient-reported outcomes 12 years after localized prostate cancer treatment. NEJM Evid. 2013;2(4) https://doi.org/10.1056/EVIDoa2300018.
24. Koeman M, Van Driel M, Weijmar Schultz W, et al. Orgasm after radical prostatectomy. Br J Urol. 1996;77:861.
25. Clavell-Hernández J, Martin C, Wang R. Orgasmic dysfunction following radical prostatectomy: review of current literature. Sex Med Rev. 2018;6:124.
26. Ganzer R, Hadaschik B, Pahernik S, et al. Prospective multicenter phase II study on focal therapy (hemiablation) of the prostate with high intensity focused ultrasound. J Urol. 2018;199:983.
27. von Hardenberg J, Westhoff N, Baumunk D, et al. Prostate cancer treatment by the latest focal HIFU device with MRI/TRUS-fusion control biopsies: a prospective evaluation. Presented at the Urologic Oncology: Seminars and Original Investigations. Urol Oncol. 2018;36(9):401.e1–9.
28. Shoji S, Hiraiwa S, Uemura K, et al. Focal therapy with high-intensity focused ultrasound for the localized prostate cancer for Asian based on the localization with MRI-TRUS fusion image-guided transperineal biopsy and 12-cores transperineal systematic biopsy: prospective analysis of oncological and functional outcomes. Int J Clin Oncol. 2020;25:1844.
29. Noweski A, Roosen A, Lebdai S, et al. Medium-term follow-up of vascular-targeted photodynamic therapy of localized prostate cancer using TOOKAD soluble WST-11 (phase II trials). Eur Urol Focus. 2019;5:1022.
30. Hopstaken JS, Bomers JGR, Sedelaar MJP, et al. An updated systematic review on focal therapy in localized prostate cancer: what has changed over the past 5 years? Eur Urol. 2022;81:5.
31. Boissier R, Sanguedolce F, Territo A, et al. Whole and hemi-gland cryoablation for primary localized prostate cancer: short and medium-term oncological and functional outcomes. Actas Urol Esp (Engl Ed). 2020;44:172.
32. Mendez MH, Passoni NM, Pow-Sang J, et al. Comparison of outcomes between preoperatively potent men treated with focal versus whole gland cryotherapy in a matched population. J Endourol. 2015;29:1193.
33. Aydin AM, Gage K, Dhillon J, et al. Focal bipolar radiofrequency ablation for localized prostate cancer: safety and feasibility. Int J Urol. 2020;27:882.
34. Orczyk C, Barratt D, Brew-Graves C, et al. Prostate radiofrequency focal ablation (ProRAFT) trial: a prospective development study evaluating a bipolar radiofrequency device to treat prostate cancer. J Urol. 2021;205:1090.
35. Faris S, Kaufman M. LUTS after radiotherapy for prostate cancer: evaluation and treatment. Curr Bladder Dysfunct Rep. 2015;10:150.
36. Alshak MN, Eidelberg A, Diaz SM, et al. Natural history of lower urinary tract symptoms among men undergoing stereotactic body radiation therapy for prostate cancer with and without a rectal hydrogel spacer. World J Urol. 2022;40:1143.
37. Venderbos LD, Deschamps A, Dowling J, et al. Europa uomo patient reported outcome study (EUPROMS): descriptive statistics of a prostate cancer survey from patients for patients. Eur Urol Focus. 2021;7:987.

The Future of Prostate Cancer Treatment 13

Dallin Busby and Mani Menon

Introduction

The advancements in surgery, radiation therapy, and medication for the treatment of prostate cancer (PCa) are remarkable accomplishments, and these innovations are a recent phenomenon. If the entire span of *Homo sapiens* existence was represented as the length of an American football field, the amount of time since the first recorded abdominal surgery would be approximately 3 inches, and the time since the first prostatectomy would be less than 2 inches [1, 2]. Years ago, the ability to perform an open radical prostatectomy (RP) was the sign of a truly competent urologic surgeon, owing to the challenge of accessing the organ that is deeply seated in the pelvis. Now, RP is regularly performed during residency training and is seen as a core surgery for urologists.

Yet, despite the remarkable progress of the last 120 years, PCa remains the most common noncutaneous cancer in men (approximately one in eight men will develop cancer in their lifetime), and mortality rates have been essentially stable for the past 10 years [3]. With an eye toward the future of PCa care, we first look back at the progress of the last 120 years.

History

Hugh Hampton Young performed the first perineal RP for PCa in 1904 with assistance from William Halstead [4, 5]. Portions of the prostate were removed for select patients with urinary retention secondary to benign prostatic hypertrophy (BPH)

D. Busby (✉) · M. Menon
Department of Urology, Icahn School of Medicine at Mount Sinai Hospital, New York, NY, USA
e-mail: Busbyd@uthscsa.edu; Mani.Menon@mountsinai.org

S. Razdan, S. Razdan (eds.), *Urinary Continence and Sexual Function After Robotic Prostatectomy, Radiation, and Novel Therapies*,
https://doi.org/10.1007/978-3-031-64245-6_13

prior to this operation, but this was the first removal of the entire prostate due to carcinoma. In 1945, Terrence Millin described the extravesical retropubic prostatectomy for BPH [6]. Shortly thereafter, several urologists began performing retropubic RP, noting that the "anatomy is less complicated" and the "operation is easier to perform" than the perineal alternative [7]. Both the perineal and retropubic approach harbored significant morbidity, including rectal injury, massive hemorrhage, pulmonary embolus, lymphocele, infection, and incontinence, with near universal impotence [8].

Expanding upon previous knowledge [9] that trauma to the sacral parasympathetic nerves during surgery interferes with erectile function, Finkle and Saunders described techniques for preserving parasympathetic nerves during perineal RP in 1960 [10]. In the early 1980s, Patrick Walsh and colleagues made several discoveries that improved outcomes for patients undergoing retropubic RP. First, he described the dorsal venous complex and a method for its ligation to decrease blood loss and improve vision of the prostate during dissection [11]. The improved vision that this step afforded made future enhancements of surgical techniques possible. He then described the innervation of the corpora cavernosum using fetal anatomic studies and concluded that impotence after RP was due to damage of these nerves [12]. In 1982, Walsh performed the first nerve-sparing RP in an effort to improve postoperative potency [13]. After the nerve-sparing RP, 5/6 (83%) of men with sexual partners who were followed for at least 6 months were fully potent [13]. This ushered in an era when the conversation shifted from "can we remove the cancer?" to "how can we provide the best functional outcomes while removing all the cancer?" Function became a consideration, and the field charged forward.

In 1991, Schuessler et al. performed the first laparoscopic RP, though this approach never gained widespread enthusiasm due to a steep learning curve and failure to demonstrate superiority over the open approach [14, 15]. After the creation of the da Vinci surgical system (Intuitive Surgical, Inc., Sunnyvale, CA), the first robotic-assisted laparoscopic radical prostatectomy (RALP) was performed in the early 2000s [16].

Present Day

Aided by the vigorous outcome tracking and reporting from Menon and colleagues at the Vattikuti Urology Institute, the RALP grew in popularity in the early 2000s, with two-thirds of RP utilizing the robotic approach by 2010 and estimates of nearly 85% in 2020. [17–20] Menon and colleagues established the first large-scale robotic prostatectomy program, devoting significant resources to vigorous outcome tracking of their early experience and demonstrating improved blood loss, postoperative pain, and early discharge when compared with the open prostatectomy cohort.

Cost-effectiveness analysis has shown that RALP is more cost-effective than laparoscopic and open RP due to improved functional outcomes, lower complication rates, and lower biochemical recurrence rates [21]. Some have argued that even though cost-effectiveness analyses provide important information, "it is time to accept robotic prostatectomy as a fixture in a urologist's armamentarium," as it is unlikely that significant portions of the field will return to open prostatectomy, even if a small economic advantage was found in favor of the open approach [22]. Recently, the advancement of the single-port robotic surgical system has enhanced the transvesical and extraperitoneal approaches to RP [23–25]. Robotic surgery has also grown in other surgical subspecialties, including gynecology, otolaryngology, cardiothoracic surgery, general surgery, and orthopedics [26].

New surgical techniques have been developed in an effort to improve functional outcomes after RP. In particular, the posterior (Retzius-sparing) approach has been shown to improve early return of continence following RP, though this difference disappears by 1 year [27–30]. Enhanced methods of nerve sparing have been shown to improve erectile function after RP [31, 32]. Finally, subtotal precision prostatectomy has been investigated as a form of focal therapy with the goal of maximizing postoperative functional status without compromising cancer control. Sood et al. described the precision prostatectomy, wherein a rim of prostatic tissue is preserved on the nondominant side of the gland to maximize nerve preservation and erectile function [33].

Future

As we look forward to the coming years of prostate surgery, there are several possibilities for the expansion of the current surgical paradigm. Currently, local radiation therapy is offered to patients with low-burden metastatic disease following the results of the STAMPEDE trial [34]. Early studies have suggested that RP may also offer survival benefits in this population, but further clinical trials are needed to evaluate this possibility [35–39]. We urge urologists to continue to strive to improve surgical outcomes by robustly tracking outcomes data. When seeking to answer a specific question, randomized controlled trials (RCTs) are reliable means to finding answers. Realistically, it is challenging to answer every question with a RCT. Collaborative quality initiatives (e.g. Michigan Urological Surgery Improvement Collaborative [MUSIC]), prospective registries, and registry-based RCTs can provide important information when RCTs are not feasible. Tracking outcomes with these processes is important to reliably assess whether surgical outcomes are improving. Nonetheless, future treatments apart from, and perhaps in conjunction with, surgery will continue to develop in the coming years.

Androgen deprivation therapy (ADT) has played a role in the treatment of men with PCa, since described by Huggins and Hodges in 1941 [40]. To overcome the eventual transition to castration resistance, recent work has investigated the use of bipolar ADT, where high doses of testosterone are given for a short amount of time, followed by ADT [41]. Early clinical trials have shown promising results and further trials are ongoing [42–44].

As personalized medicine advances, the genetic and molecular characteristics of an individual patients' cancer may be able to be targeted with novel treatments to enhance survival. For example, PARP inhibitors [45, 46], androgen receptor inhibitors [47, 48], and checkpoint inhibitors [49, 50] have been shown to improve survival for patients with advanced disease, though these improvements are only marginal [51]. With increased availability of genetic testing for men diagnosed with PCa, additional therapeutic targets may emerge.

Immunotherapy is another developing treatment for PCa. Immunotherapy involves using the immune system to recognize and attack cancer cells. Immune checkpoint inhibitors [52], therapeutic cancer vaccines [53], and T cell engineering [54, 55] are some examples of immunotherapeutic approaches for the treatment of PCa. As the field of immunotherapy grows, its role in the treatment of PCa may expand [56].

Prostate-specific membrane antigen (PSMA) has been leveraged for PCa, staging with PET/CT imaging [57]. Additionally, the utilization of PSMA-radioligands during surgery may help increase the yield of lymph node dissection by identifying nodal metastasis outside of the extended lymph node dissection template [58]. In time, similar techniques may be used to help improve nerve preservation without increasing positive margin rates if used during the nerve-sparing stage of RALP. Additionally, early studies have shown the benefit of endoradiotherapy with lutetium-177-PSMA-617 in men with advanced diseases, but further randomized trials are needed to fully assess this treatment [59, 60].

Focal therapy for primary localized PCa is also an emerging treatment option. To date, the American Urological Association (AUA) and European Association of Urology (EAU) both state that there is insufficient evidence to recommend focal therapy as a treatment option while encouraging prospective trial development [61, 62]. Systematic reviews have generally shown that functional outcomes after focal therapy are improved relative to whole-gland treatment, but oncologic results varied and hard to characterize [63–67].

Finally, as the reach of artificial intelligence (AI) has expanded in many sectors of society, PCa treatment has also incorporated AI. Artificial intelligence has been used for PCa risk stratification for many years [68, 69], but more recently, it has been used to help with radiographic detection [70], histopathologic diagnosis [71], assessment of surgeon competency [72], and prediction of surgical outcomes [73]. Taken together, these applications of AI show that technology can be leveraged to improve PCa care across many domains.

Conclusion

For years, the retropubic RP was thought to be the most challenging operation in urology, and many of the leaders in the field were known for the advancements they pioneered. With the spread of robotic surgery, many urologists now routinely perform RALP. Beginning with Patrick Walsh in 1982, the focus for PCa surgery has been achieving the best functional results while safely removing the cancer. In the early 2000s, urologists paved the way into the future of surgery by embracing robotic surgery. In the coming years, additional therapies will continue to emerge, which may enhance or detract from the role of surgery. Let us continue to push forward as we treat PCa in a patient-centered manner.

Take-Home Message
The future of prostate cancer treatment involves the interplay of precision surgery, personalized medicine, targeted pharmaceuticals, and focal therapies. The urologist will have numerous surgical and nonsurgical options to treat men with prostate cancer while continuing to advance urinary continence and erectile function outcomes.

References

1. Hublin JJ, Ben-Ncer A, Bailey SE, et al. New fossils from Jebel Irhoud, Morocco and the pan-African origin of Homo sapiens. Nature. 2017;546(7657):289–92. https://doi.org/10.1038/nature22336.
2. Marcy HO. The early history of abdominal surgery in America. JAMA J Am Med Assoc. 1910;LIV(8):600–5. https://doi.org/10.1001/jama.1910.92550340001001f.
3. Siegel RL, Miller KD, Wagle NS, Jemal A. Cancer statistics, 2023. CA Cancer J Clin. 2023;73(1):17–48. https://doi.org/10.3322/caac.21763.
4. VIII YHH. Conservative perineal prostatectomy: the results of two years' experience and report of seventy-five cases. Ann Surg. 1905;41(4):549–57.
5. Young HH. The early diagnosis and radical cure of carcinoma of the prostate. Being a study of 40 cases and presentation of a radical operation which was carried out in four cases. 1905. J Urol. 2002;168(3):914–21. https://doi.org/10.1016/s0022-5347(05)64542-9.
6. Millin T. Retropubic prostatectomy; a new extravesical technique; report of 20 cases. Lancet. 1945;2(6380):693–6. https://doi.org/10.1016/s0140-6736(45)91030-0.
7. Chute R. Radical retropubic prostatectomy for cancer. J Urol. 1954;71(3):347–72. https://doi.org/10.1016/s0022-5347(17)67796-6.
8. Lepor H. A review of surgical techniques for radical prostatectomy. Rev Urol. 2005;7 Suppl 2(Suppl 2):S11–7.
9. Morgan JW, Saunders JB de CM. Preservation of genito-urinary function in rectal resection. Proc R Soc Med. 1950;43(12):1081–3.
10. Finkle AL, Saunders JB. Sexual potency in aging males. III. Technic of avoiding nerve injury in perineal prostatic operations. Am J Surg. 1960;99:23–6. https://doi.org/10.1016/0002-9610(60)90243-9.
11. Reiner WG, Walsh PC. An anatomical approach to the surgical management of the dorsal vein and Santorini's plexus during radical retropubic surgery. J Urol. 1979;121(2):198–200. https://doi.org/10.1016/s0022-5347(17)56718-x.
12. Walsh PC, Donker PJ. Impotence following radical prostatectomy: insight into etiology and prevention. J Urol. 1982;128(3):492–7. https://doi.org/10.1016/S0022-5347(17)53012-8.
13. Walsh PC, Lepor H, Eggleston JC. Radical prostatectomy with preservation of sexual function: anatomical and pathological considerations. Prostate. 1983;4(5):473–85. https://doi.org/10.1002/pros.2990040506.
14. Schuessler WW, Schulam PG, Clayman RV, Kavoussi LR. Laparoscopic radical prostatectomy: initial short-term experience. Urology. 1997;50(6):854–7. https://doi.org/10.1016/S0090-4295(97)00543-8.
15. Shuford MD. Robotically assisted laparoscopic radical prostatectomy: a brief review of outcomes. Proc (Baylor Univ Med Cent). 2007;20(4):354–6. https://doi.org/10.1080/08998280.2007.11928322.

16. Pasticier G, Rietbergen JB, Guillonneau B, Fromont G, Menon M, Vallancien G. Robotically assisted laparoscopic radical prostatectomy: feasibility study in men. Eur Urol. 2001;40(1):70–4. https://doi.org/10.1159/000049751.
17. Menon M, Tewari A, Vattikuti Institute Prostatectomy Team. Robotic radical prostatectomy and the Vattikuti urology institute technique: an interim analysis of results and technical points. Urology. 2003;61(4 Suppl 1):15–20. https://doi.org/10.1016/s0090-4295(03)00116-x.
18. Menon M, Tewari A, Baize B, Guillonneau B, Vallancien G. Prospective comparison of radical retropubic prostatectomy and robot-assisted anatomic prostatectomy: the Vattikuti Urology Institute experience. Urology. 2002;60(5):864–8. https://doi.org/10.1016/s0090-4295(02)01881-2.
19. Lowrance WT, Eastham JA, Savage C, et al. Contemporary open and robotic radical prostatectomy practice patterns among urologists in the United States. J Urol. 2012;187(6):2087–92. https://doi.org/10.1016/j.juro.2012.01.061.
20. Crew B. Worth the cost? A closer look at the da Vinci robot's impact on prostate cancer surgery. Nature. 2020;580(7804):S5–7. https://doi.org/10.1038/d41586-020-01037-w.
21. Labban M, Dasgupta P, Song C, et al. Cost-effectiveness of robotic-assisted radical prostatectomy for localized prostate cancer in the UK. JAMA Netw Open. 2022;5(4):e225740. https://doi.org/10.1001/jamanetworkopen.2022.5740.
22. Golla V, Williams SB. Cost-effectiveness of robotic-assisted prostatectomy in the UK-are we doing enough? JAMA Netw Open. 2022;5(4):e225747. https://doi.org/10.1001/jamanetworkopen.2022.5747.
23. Kaouk J, Beksac AT, Abou Zeinab M, Duncan A, Schwen ZR, Eltemamy M. Single port Transvesical robotic radical prostatectomy: initial clinical experience and description of technique. Urology. 2021;155:130–7. https://doi.org/10.1016/j.urology.2021.05.022.
24. Kaouk J, Valero R, Sawczyn G, Garisto J. Extraperitoneal single-port robot-assisted radical prostatectomy: initial experience and description of technique. BJU Int. 2020;125(1):182–9. https://doi.org/10.1111/bju.14885.
25. Lai A, Dobbs RW, Talamini S, et al. Single port robotic radical prostatectomy: a systematic review. Transl Androl Urol. 2020;9(2):898–905. https://doi.org/10.21037/tau.2019.11.05.
26. Shah J, Vyas A, Vyas D. The History of robotics in surgical specialties. Am J Robot Surg. 2014;1(1):12–20. https://doi.org/10.1166/ajrs.2014.1006.
27. Galfano A, Ascione A, Grimaldi S, Petralia G, Strada E, Bocciardi AM. A new anatomic approach for robot-assisted laparoscopic prostatectomy: a feasibility study for completely intrafascial surgery. Eur Urol. 2010;58(3):457–61. https://doi.org/10.1016/j.eururo.2010.06.008.
28. Rosenberg JE, Jung JH, Edgerton Z, et al. Retzius-sparing versus standard robotic-assisted laparoscopic prostatectomy for the treatment of clinically localized prostate cancer. Cochrane Database Syst Rev. 2020;8:CD013641. https://doi.org/10.1002/14651858.CD013641.pub2.
29. Dalela D, Jeong W, Prasad MA, et al. A pragmatic randomized controlled trial examining the impact of the Retzius-sparing approach on early urinary continence recovery after robot-assisted radical prostatectomy. Eur Urol. 2017;72(5):677–85. https://doi.org/10.1016/j.eururo.2017.04.029.
30. Menon M, Dalela D, Jamil M, et al. Functional recovery, oncologic outcomes and postoperative complications after robot-assisted radical prostatectomy: an evidence-based analysis comparing the Retzius sparing and standard approaches. J Urol. 2018;199(5):1210–7. https://doi.org/10.1016/j.juro.2017.11.115.
31. Kaul S, Savera A, Badani K, Fumo M, Bhandari A, Menon M. Functional outcomes and oncological efficacy of Vattikuti institute prostatectomy with Veil of Aphrodite nerve-sparing: an analysis of 154 consecutive patients. BJU Int. 2006;97(3):467–72. https://doi.org/10.1111/j.1464-410X.2006.05990.x.
32. Wagaskar VG, Mittal A, Sobotka S, et al. Hood technique for robotic radical prostatectomy-preserving periurethral anatomical structures in the space of Retzius and sparing the pouch of Douglas, enabling early return of continence without compromising surgical margin rates. Eur Urol. 2021;80(2):213–21. https://doi.org/10.1016/j.eururo.2020.09.044.

33. Sood A, Jeong W, Palma-Zamora I, et al. Description of surgical technique and oncologic and functional outcomes of the precision prostatectomy procedure (IDEAL stage 1–2b study). Eur Urol. 2022;81(4):396–406. https://doi.org/10.1016/j.eururo.2021.10.017.
34. Parker CC, James ND, Brawley CD, et al. Radiotherapy to the primary tumour for newly diagnosed, metastatic prostate cancer (STAMPEDE): a randomised controlled phase 3 trial. Lancet. 2018;392(10162):2353–66. https://doi.org/10.1016/S0140-6736(18)32486-3.
35. Mandel P, Steuber T, Graefen M. Radical prostatectomy in oligometastatic prostate cancer. Curr Opin Urol. 2017;27(6):572–9. https://doi.org/10.1097/MOU.0000000000000445.
36. Leyh-Bannurah SR, Gazdovich S, Budäus L, et al. Local therapy improves survival in metastatic prostate cancer. Eur Urol. 2017;72(1):118–24. https://doi.org/10.1016/j.eururo.2017.03.020.
37. Yuh BE, Kwon YS, Shinder BM, et al. Results of phase 1 study on cytoreductive radical prostatectomy in men with newly diagnosed metastatic prostate cancer. Prostate Int. 2019;7(3):102–7. https://doi.org/10.1016/j.prnil.2018.10.002.
38. Dai B, Zhang S, Wan FN, et al. Combination of androgen deprivation therapy with radical local therapy versus androgen deprivation therapy alone for newly diagnosed Oligometastatic prostate cancer: a phase II randomized controlled trial. Eur Urol Oncol. 2022;5(5):519–25. https://doi.org/10.1016/j.euo.2022.06.001.
39. Rajwa P, Zattoni F, Maggi M, et al. Cytoreductive radical prostatectomy for metastatic hormone-sensitive prostate cancer-evidence from recent prospective reports. *Eur Urol Focus*. Published online January 23, 2023:S2405-4569(23)00024-X. https://doi.org/10.1016/j.euf.2023.01.011.
40. Huggins C, Hodges CV. Studies on prostatic cancer. I. The effect of castration, of estrogen and androgen injection on serum phosphatases in metastatic carcinoma of the prostate. Cancer Res. 1941;1:293–7.
41. Denmeade SR, Isaacs JT. Bipolar androgen therapy: the rationale for rapid cycling of supraphysiologic androgen/ablation in men with castration resistant prostate cancer. Prostate. 2010;70(14):1600–7. https://doi.org/10.1002/pros.21196.
42. Teply BA, Wang H, Luber B, et al. Bipolar androgen therapy in men with metastatic castration-resistant prostate cancer after progression on enzalutamide: an open-label, phase 2, multicohort study. Lancet Oncol. 2018;19(1):76–86. https://doi.org/10.1016/S1470-2045(17)30906-3.
43. Markowski MC, Wang H, Sullivan R, et al. A multicohort open-label phase II trial of bipolar androgen therapy in men with metastatic castration-resistant prostate cancer (RESTORE): a comparison of post-abiraterone versus post-enzalutamide cohorts. Eur Urol. 2021;79(5):692–9. https://doi.org/10.1016/j.eururo.2020.06.042.
44. Denmeade SR, Wang H, Agarwal N, et al. TRANSFORMER: a randomized phase II study comparing bipolar androgen therapy versus enzalutamide in asymptomatic men with castration-resistant metastatic prostate cancer. J Clin Oncol. 2021;39(12):1371–82. https://doi.org/10.1200/JCO.20.02759.
45. Mateo J, Porta N, Bianchini D, et al. Olaparib in patients with metastatic castration-resistant prostate cancer with DNA repair gene aberrations (TOPARP-B): a multicentre, open-label, randomised, phase 2 trial. Lancet Oncol. 2020;21(1):162–74. https://doi.org/10.1016/S1470-2045(19)30684-9.
46. Abida W, Patnaik A, Campbell D, et al. Rucaparib in men with metastatic castration-resistant prostate cancer harboring a BRCA1 or BRCA2 gene alteration. J Clin Oncol. 2020;38(32):3763–72. https://doi.org/10.1200/JCO.20.01035.
47. Scher HI, Fizazi K, Saad F, et al. Increased survival with enzalutamide in prostate cancer after chemotherapy. N Engl J Med. 2012;367(13):1187–97. https://doi.org/10.1056/NEJMoa1207506.
48. Ryan CJ, Smith MR, Fizazi K, et al. Abiraterone acetate plus prednisone versus placebo plus prednisone in chemotherapy-naive men with metastatic castration-resistant prostate cancer (COU-AA-302): final overall survival analysis of a randomised, double-blind, placebo-controlled phase 3 study. Lancet Oncol. 2015;16(2):152–60. https://doi.org/10.1016/S1470-2045(14)71205-7.

49. Sharma P, Retz M, Siefker-Radtke A, et al. Nivolumab in metastatic urothelial carcinoma after platinum therapy (CheckMate 275): a multicentre, single-arm, phase 2 trial. Lancet Oncol. 2017;18(3):312–22. https://doi.org/10.1016/S1470-2045(17)30065-7.
50. Antonarakis ES, Piulats JM, Gross-Goupil M, et al. Pembrolizumab for treatment-refractory metastatic castration-resistant prostate cancer: multicohort, open-label phase II KEYNOTE-199 study. J Clin Oncol. 2020;38(5):395–405. https://doi.org/10.1200/JCO.19.01638.
51. Kim IE, Jang TL, Kim S, et al. Marginal improvement in survival among patients diagnosed with metastatic prostate cancer in the second-line antiandrogen therapy era. Cancer Med. 2021;10(22):7909–20. https://doi.org/10.1002/cam4.4074.
52. Venkatachalam S, McFarland TR, Agarwal N, Swami U. Immune checkpoint inhibitors in prostate cancer. Cancers (Basel). 2021;13(9):2187. https://doi.org/10.3390/cancers13092187.
53. Kantoff PW, Higano CS, Shore ND, et al. Sipuleucel-T immunotherapy for castration-resistant prostate cancer. N Engl J Med. 2010;363(5):411–22. https://doi.org/10.1056/NEJMoa1001294.
54. Sadelain M, Rivière I, Riddell S. Therapeutic T cell engineering. Nature. 2017;545(7655):423–31. https://doi.org/10.1038/nature22395.
55. Kloss CC, Lee J, Zhang A, et al. Dominant-negative TGF-β receptor enhances PSMA-targeted human CAR T cell proliferation and augments prostate cancer eradication. Mol Ther. 2018;26(7):1855–66. https://doi.org/10.1016/j.ymthe.2018.05.003.
56. Cha HR, Lee JH, Ponnazhagan S. Revisiting immunotherapy: a focus on prostate cancer. Cancer Res. 2020;80(8):1615–23. https://doi.org/10.1158/0008-5472.CAN-19-2948.
57. National Comprehensive Cancer Network. Prostate cancer (version 4.2022). NCCN. Accessed 27 May 2022. https://www.nccn.org/guidelines/guidelines-detail
58. Lunger L, Steinhelfer L, Korn P, et al. Prostate-specific membrane antigen-radioguided surgery facilitates pelvic lymph node dissection during radical prostatectomy for the treatment of locally advanced prostate cancer with regional lymph node metastases. Eur Urol Oncol. 2023;6(1):95–8. https://doi.org/10.1016/j.euo.2022.12.001.
59. Hofman MS, Violet J, Hicks RJ, et al. [177Lu]-PSMA-617 radionuclide treatment in patients with metastatic castration-resistant prostate cancer (LuPSMA trial): a single-centre, single-arm, phase 2 study. Lancet Oncol. 2018;19(6):825–33. https://doi.org/10.1016/S1470-2045(18)30198-0.
60. Sadaghiani MS, Sheikhbahaei S, Werner RA, et al. A systematic review and meta-analysis of the effectiveness and toxicities of lutetium-177-labeled prostate-specific membrane antigen-targeted radioligand therapy in metastatic castration-resistant prostate cancer. Eur Urol. 2021;80(1):82–94. https://doi.org/10.1016/j.eururo.2021.03.004.
61. Eastham JA, Auffenberg GB, Barocas DA, et al. Clinically localized prostate cancer: AUA/ASTRO guideline, part I: introduction, risk assessment, staging, and risk-based management. J Urol. 2022;208(1):10–8. https://doi.org/10.1097/JU.0000000000002757.
62. EAU Guidelines. Presented at the EAU annual congress. Amsterdam; 2022.
63. Hopstaken JS, Bomers JGR, Sedelaar MJP, Valerio M, Fütterer JJ, Rovers MM. An updated systematic review on focal therapy in localized prostate cancer: what has changed over the past 5 years? Eur Urol. 2022;81(1):5–33. https://doi.org/10.1016/j.eururo.2021.08.005.
64. Bates AS, Ayers J, Kostakopoulos N, et al. A systematic review of focal ablative therapy for clinically localised prostate cancer in comparison with standard management options: limitations of the available evidence and recommendations for clinical practice and further research. Eur Urol Oncol. 2021;4(3):405–23. https://doi.org/10.1016/j.euo.2020.12.008.
65. Valerio M, Ahmed HU, Emberton M, et al. The role of focal therapy in the management of localised prostate cancer: a systematic review. Eur Urol. 2014;66(4):732–51. https://doi.org/10.1016/j.eururo.2013.05.048.
66. Faure Walker NA, Norris JM, Shah TT, et al. A comparison of time taken to return to baseline erectile function following focal and whole gland ablative therapies for localized prostate cancer: a systematic review. Urol Oncol. 2018;36(2):67–76. https://doi.org/10.1016/j.urolonc.2017.12.002.

67. Fiard G, Chowdhury A, Potter AR, et al. Detailing sexual outcomes after focal therapy for localised prostate cancer: a systematic review and meta-analysis. Eur Urol Focus. Published online September 24, 2021:S2405-4569(21)00238-8. https://doi.org/10.1016/j.euf.2021.09.009.
68. Tewari A, Narayan P. Novel staging tool for localized prostate cancer: a pilot study using genetic adaptive neural networks. J Urol. 1998;160(2):430–6. https://doi.org/10.1016/s0022-5347(01)62916-1.
69. Cordon-Cardo C, Kotsianti A, Verbel DA, et al. Improved prediction of prostate cancer recurrence through systems pathology. J Clin Invest. 2007;117(7):1876–83. https://doi.org/10.1172/JCI31399.
70. Giganti F, Panebianco V, Tempany CM, Purysko AS. Is artificial intelligence replacing our radiology stars in prostate magnetic resonance imaging? The stars do not look big, but they can look brighter. Eur Urol Open Sci. 2023;48:12–3. https://doi.org/10.1016/j.euros.2022.11.021.
71. Busby D, Grauer R, Pandav K, et al. Applications of artificial intelligence in prostate cancer histopathology. Urol Oncol. Published online January 11, 2023:S1078-1439(22)00487-2. https://doi.org/10.1016/j.urolonc.2022.12.002.
72. Hung AJ, Chen J, Gill IS. Automated performance metrics and machine learning algorithms to measure surgeon performance and anticipate clinical outcomes in robotic surgery. JAMA Surg. 2018;153(8):770–1. https://doi.org/10.1001/jamasurg.2018.1512.
73. Trinh L, Mingo S, Vanstrum EB, et al. Survival analysis using surgeon skill metrics and patient factors to predict urinary continence recovery after robot-assisted radical prostatectomy. Eur Urol Focus. 2022;8(2):623–30. https://doi.org/10.1016/j.euf.2021.04.001.

Correction to: Imaging Modalities for Prostate Cancer

Hala Khasawneh, Dina Hamdan,
and Pamela Causa Andrieu

Correction to:
Chapter 2 in: S. Razdan, S. Razdan (eds.),
Urinary Continence and Sexual Function After Robotic Prostatectomy, Radiation, and Novel Therapies,
https://doi.org/10.1007/978-3-031-64245-6_2

The book was inadvertently published with an incorrect spelling of the author's name in Chap. 2 as Dinna Hamdan, whereas it should be Dina Hamdan.

The updated version of this chapter can be found at
https://doi.org/10.1007/978-3-031-64245-6_2

S. Razdan, S. Razdan (eds.), *Urinary Continence and Sexual Function After Robotic Prostatectomy, Radiation, and Novel Therapies*,
https://doi.org/10.1007/978-3-031-64245-6_14

Index

S. Razdan, S. Razdan (eds.), *Urinary Continence and Sexual Function After Robotic Prostatectomy, Radiation, and Novel Therapies*, https://doi.org/10.1007/978-3-031-64245-6

L

M

N